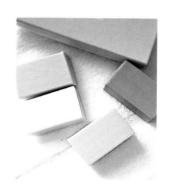

zest ●

weekend ○

home ○

spa ●

zest

week

ho

end me Spa

LINDA BIRD

NEW HOLLAND

Published in 2001 by
New Holland Publishers (UK) Ltd
London • Cape Town • Sydney • Auckland

Garfield House
86 Edgware Road
London W2 2EA
United Kingdom

80 McKenzie Street
Cape Town 8001
South Africa

Level 1, Unit 4, 14 Aquatic Drive
Frenchs Forest, NSW 2086
Australia

218 Lake Road
Northcote, Auckland
New Zealand

ISBN 1 85974 618 7

Editor: Louisa Somerville
Picture research: Sarah Moule
Production: Caroline Hansell
Design: Roger Hammond
Editorial direction: Rosemary Wilkinson

10 9 8 7 6 5 4 3 2 1

Reproduction by
Modern Age Repro House Ltd, Hong Kong
Printed and bound in Singapore by
Star Standard Industries (Pte)

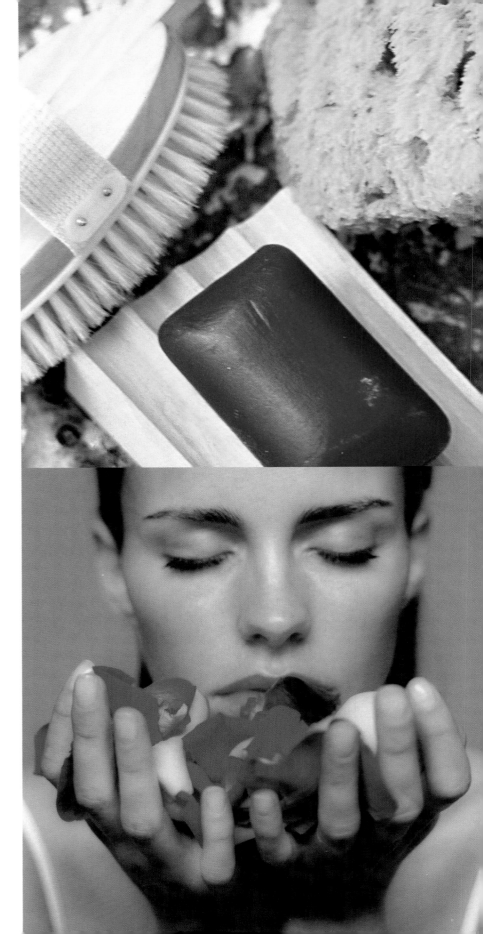

contents

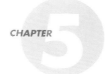

introduction

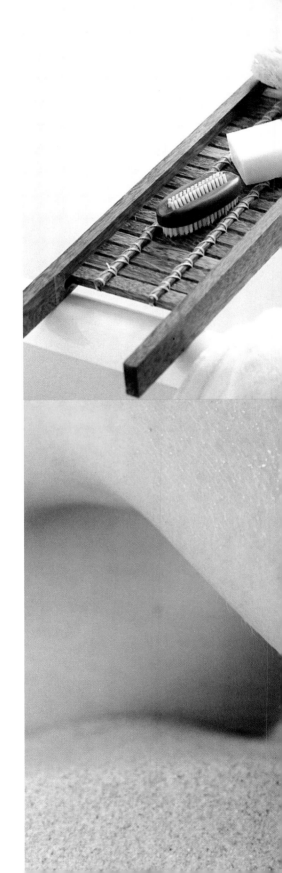

THIS BOOK IS FOR EVERY WOMAN who values her health, looks and wellbeing and is prepared to invest in them, even if her time and resources are limited. All it takes is one weekend at home. This book is not about lettuce fasts and face packs. It does not prescribe a Spartan detox or promise an unrealistic new you in just 48 hours. There are no rigid timetables to follow or long lists of potions to apply. What the book offers is simple, realistic, practical and motivating information, whether you want to cleanse and purify, energize, relax or shamelessly pamper yourself.

The **Zest Weekend Home Spa** provides you with a holistic approach to overhauling yourself – mind, body and soul – in one weekend. As well as luxurious body, skin and hair treatments, there is practical nutrition advice with easy menus to follow to help blitz your digestive system and revitalize your body. You can follow just one of the spa treatments in a weekend or combine elements from each of them to make a plan to suit your needs.

As exercise is central to any well-being programme, there are step-by-step mini workouts and wonderfully relaxing stretching routines. To ensure that your mind gets the same attention as your body during your spa weekend, there are meditation techniques and visualization processes, as well as more challenging exercises to boost your mental potential. Naturally, there are also several indulgent, beautifying rituals plus a tempting array of ingenious shortcuts to instant glamour.

Do not expect miracles. But do expect to look and feel brighter, fresher, more alert and glowing even after one weekend. Who knows, you may just find it gives you the motivation and inspiration you need to change the way you look after yourself for ever...

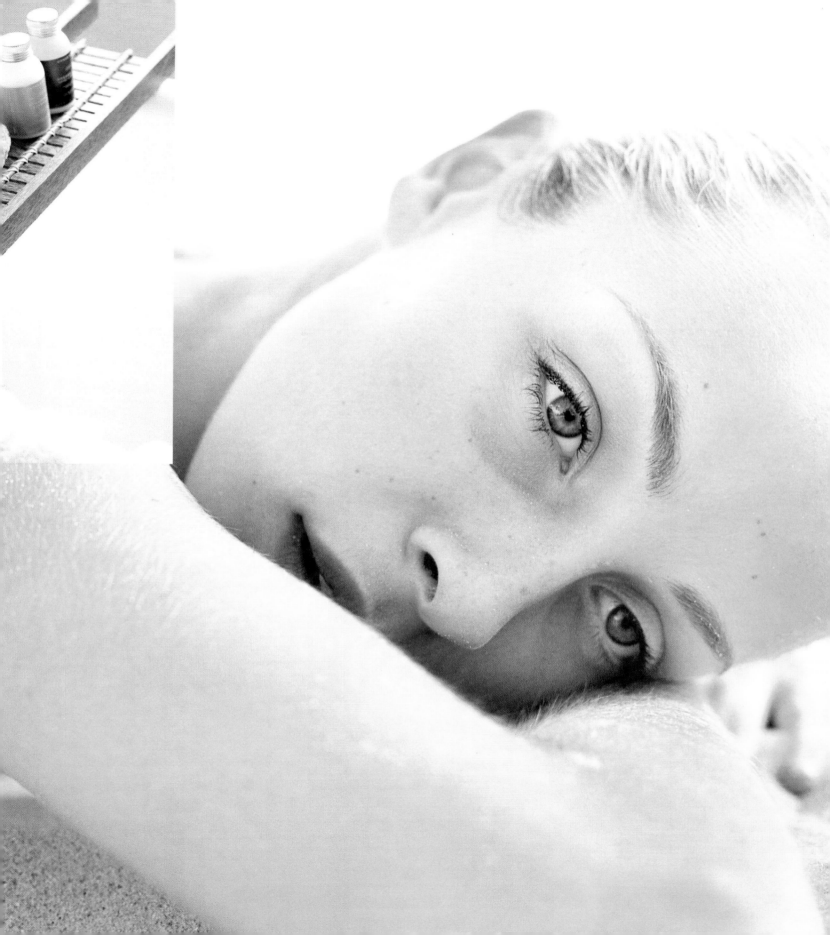

CHAPTER 1

preparation

how are you feeling? Really feeling? Many of us need a little extra sleep, less stress, more fruit and vegetables and regular exercise – all text book stuff when it comes to looking and feeling our best. However, even if you already follow a meticulous beauty routine, and work out fanatically, do you really feel truly amazing? All the time?

The truth is that daily health hazards, such as stress, lack of rest and poor nutrition, can spoil even the most strictly-observed beauty regime. What use are costly moisturizers if you seldom sleep more than five hours each night? In spite of extraordinary advances in medicine, reams of

health advice, and shelves of futuristic anti-ageing beauty treatments, time pressures and commitments – not to mention pollution – often conspire against us.

Your weekend spa is an opportunity to redress the balance. It is your chance to devote time to your own wellbeing – to sleep, to eat well and rehydrate yourself, to invigorate your body with exercise or unwind with gentle stretches and meditation. It is also designed to allow you to cover yourself head to foot with delicious unguents and envelop yourself in your favourite smells. It is a totally selfish weekend.

And you will love it.

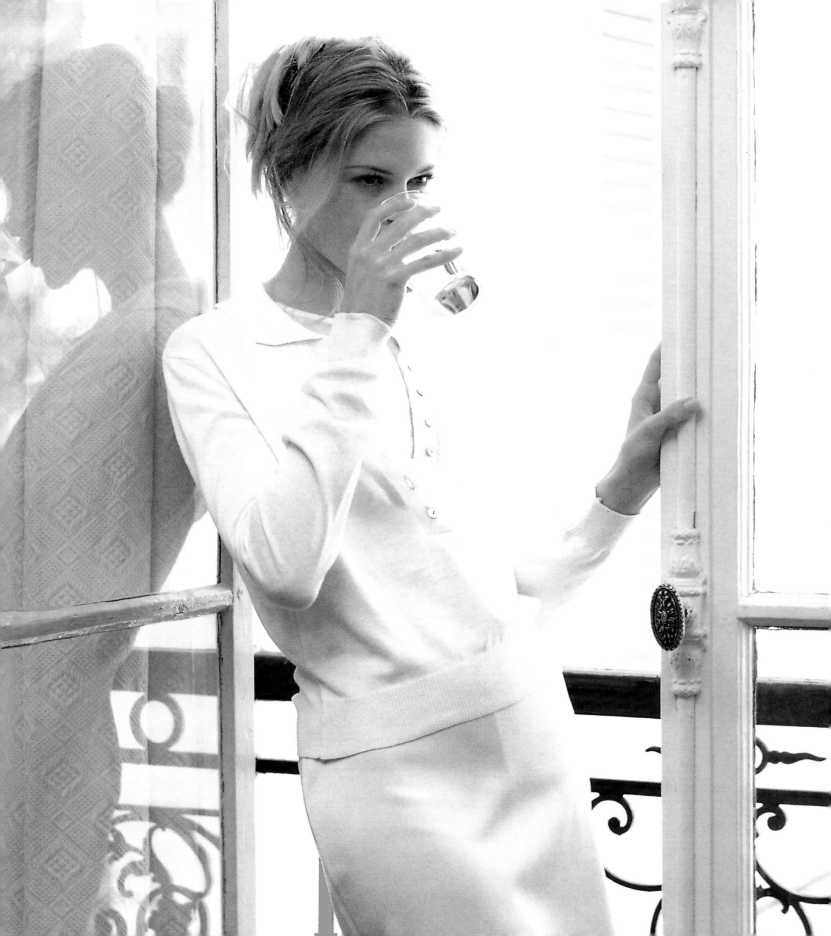

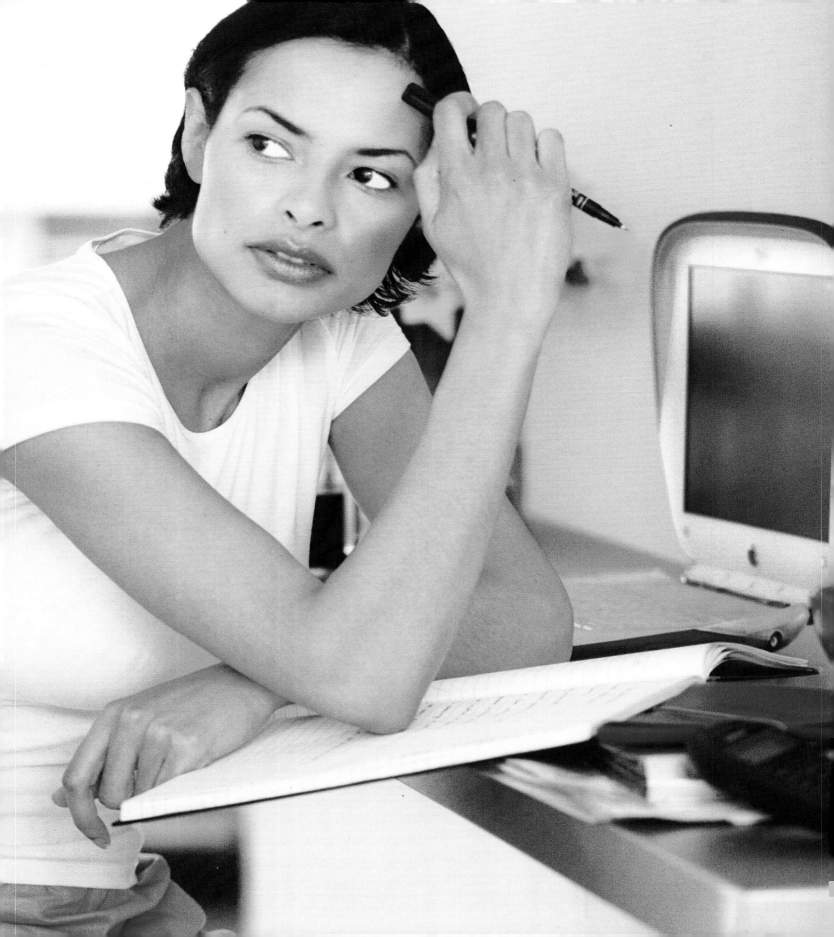

reassess your lifestyle

a face pack and an aromatherapy bath may paper over the cracks, but they are not sufficient to restore vitality. In order to derive the greatest benefit from a weekend spa, it is important to take a holistic approach to wellbeing. Take a look at your lifestyle. What may be robbing you of your vitality?

Stress

Few of us escape the effects of stress. Surveys continue to demonstrate the effect that stress has in the workplace, and women, it seems, are the most beleaguered of all: over 50 percent of us claim to suffer from stress. The repercussions on our health and wellbeing, can range from insomnia, digestive disorders, headaches and muscle tension, to lowered immunity, resulting in more coughs, colds and infections. Doctors warn that severe, prolonged stress can lead to more serious problems including post-viral fatigue and even heart disease.

Most of us notice that our skin tends to be one of the first casualties of stress. Dermatologists explain that emotional stress creates a 'fight or flight' response in the body which can starve the skin of its blood supply.

Shallow breathing, which also accompanies stress, results in cells not receiving the optimum level of oxygen required to keep them healthy, and can hasten the ageing process. Your hair too, can become dry and lacklustre in times of stress: Weight gain (or loss) is another common side effect of too much pressure.

Sleep shortage

Working too hard and relaxing too little can disrupt sleep patterns, leaving the body exhausted and prone to illness. A third of the population is said to claim difficulty in sleeping at some time in any one year. Sleep deprivation (the normal amount is six to ten hours a night) is known to depress the immune system. This leaves the body stressed and vulnerable to infection.

Our skin undergoes specific physiological processes when we sleep. The cell division that regenerates our skin, blood and brain cells increases by between 200 and 300 percent, reaching a peak at 1am. After a good night's sleep, our skin recovers elasticity and becomes more radiant. Without sleep we would find ourselves ageing very quickly.

So, to be at our mental, physical and dermatological best we ought to be clocking up a minimum of six hours each night. Few people are able to cope well on four or five hours sleep, nor should any of us be trying to.

Lack of exercise

If we don't exercise, every aspect of our wellbeing is affected. Exercise is not simply a distraction from the day's events, it is also an effective stress reliever and energy booster. Studies show that walking and running can reduce anxiety, and increase tolerance to everyday stress. Little wonder that adults are now advised to exercise for at least 30 minutes for five days a week.

When you start moving, all sorts of amazing physiological adaptations take place. Your metabolic rate increases and your body temperature rises; the increased blood flow transports more oxygen around the body, stimulating toxin drainage through the lymphatic system, helping eliminate waste products from the muscles. Collagen production increases, resulting in a thicker dermis and smoother skin.

Exercise also makes you feel good. The reason for this is the body's natural opiates, called endorphins, which are released during exercise and which block pain receptors and give the body a feeling of euphoria.

Add to that the glow that increased blood flow contributes to your skin, plus the calorie-burning power of exercise and you have one of the most effective, yet inexpensive, beauty treatments known to man.

Bad diet

Are you getting enough fruit and veg? Five portions of fruit and vegetables daily are recommended, to ensure you receive an adequate vitamin and mineral intake. Fruit and vegetables also contain anti-oxidants, which are part of the body's defence system against free radicals – molecules in the body that can damage healthy cells.

Do you drink the daily 1.5 litres (2½ pints) of water experts advise? Consistently not drinking enough adversely affects energy levels, can eventually dull the complexion, and, over prolonged periods, may lead to constipation, bladder infections and kidney stones.

A balanced diet means eating plenty of carbohydrates (such as potatoes, bread and pasta), some protein (such as meat and fish) and not much fat and sugar. It is a fact that overwork, partying or sheer apathy can all too often divert us from the right nutritional path. A poor diet can not only deplete energy levels and impair immune function, it can wreak havoc on skin and hair. The right foodstuffs, however, have the power to relax the body, promote sleep, energize, cleanse and heal. Food is indeed medicine – but it is also a useful beauty tool.

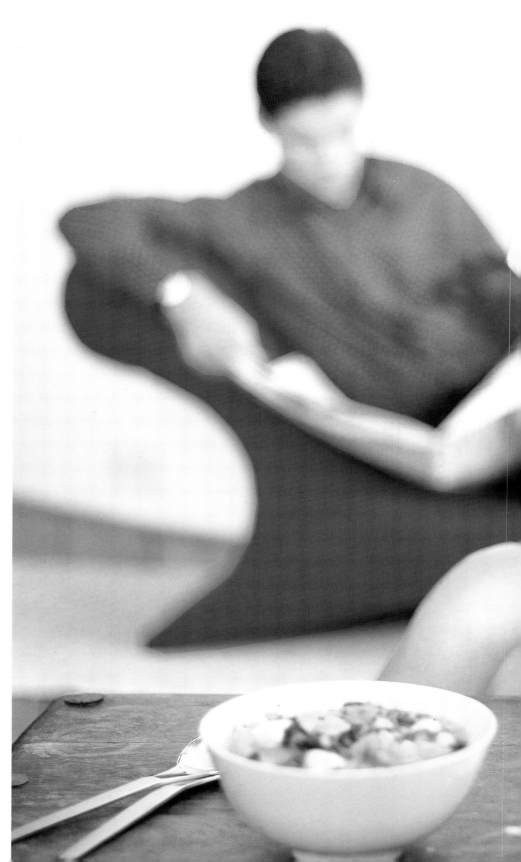

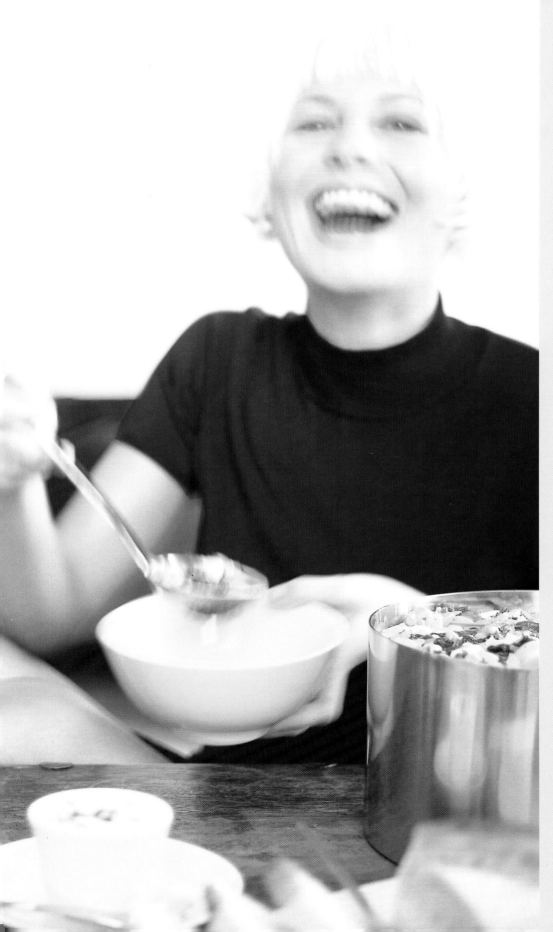

choosing the right spa

Are you ready for a refreshing, replenishing weekend spa? You may not be able to remedy downright neglect in one weekend, but a lot can be achieved. Simply eating properly, moving more, sleeping better and fretting less can change the way you look and feel.

The four principle spa programmes – the Cleansing Spa, the Energizing Spa, the Relaxation Spa and the Pampering Spa – give you the chance to take yourself in hand and get the rest, the stimulation, the nourishment and the cosseting that your body needs.

Choose a spa to restore you to your most sparkling self. Perhaps you need a thorough cleanse and polish, inside and out? Then try the Cleansing Spa. Are you in need of an energy boost? Choose the Energizing Spa. Are your body and soul crying out for a spell of idleness and relaxation? Treat yourself to a Relaxation Spa. Alternatively, if you are already fit, rested and sufficiently well nourished, you may simply enjoy a hedonistic weekend of dousing yourself in oils and lotions, champagne in hand, in the Pampering Spa.

The choice is yours.

personal consultation

Spas and health farms give their clients an assessment to ascertain their spa needs. If you are finding it difficult to work out which of our four spas will do you the most good, the following simple questionnaire may help you to plan your weekend.

1 How would describe your usual stress levels?

a) average – I work hard, but allow myself relaxation time
b) fairly low – manageable
c) very high – I often miss meals, and rely on stimulants such as coffee, cigarettes and alcohol to help me unwind
d) high – I'm always on the go

2 What is the quality of your sleep, generally?

a) deep – I find it easy to sleep and rarely wake up during the night
b) erratic – I never seem to get to bed before midnight
c) disturbed – when I have things on my mind I find it difficult to sleep
d) usually good – but I've been burning the candle at both ends recently

3 How often do you exercise?

a) regularly – I work out three or four times a week
b) rarely – I have a pretty sedentary lifestyle
c) I can't remember the last time I exercised!
d) quite good – I try to squeeze in my workout however busy I am

4 How would you describe your eating habits?

a) good – I eat well, have plenty of water and drink alcohol only occasionally
b) fairly balanced with the odd treat
c) not good at the moment – too much alcohol and fast food!
d) fairly good – but I drink a lot of coffee and/or alcohol

5 How would you describe your beauty routine?

a) thorough – I have all the latest lotions and potions
b) quite good – but I need a bit of an overhaul
c) erratic – I've let myself go a bit recently
d) it's good – when I've got the time and motivation

6 What are your main beauty concerns?

a) I want to look ultra glamorous
b) my skin and hair could do with a boost
c) I need a quick fix – from top to toe
d) I wish I had time for beauty concerns!

7 How would you describe your current state of mind?

a) good – life is good
b) I don't feel very motivated these days
c) not good – things have been getting on top of me
d) chaotic – I have so many things to worry about

Results: To find the most rewarding way to spend your weekend, add up the number of As, Bs, Cs and Ds you scored.

Mostly A Your nutrition and fitness are beyond reproach. Treat yourself to a Pampering Spa – you deserve it.
Mostly B You probably need to boost your vitality levels with the Energizing Spa.
Mostly C You've been bombarding your system with toxins. It's time for a thorough spring clean. Choose the Cleansing Spa.
Mostly D You really need to take things easy and unwind. The Relaxation Spa would give you a much-needed rest.

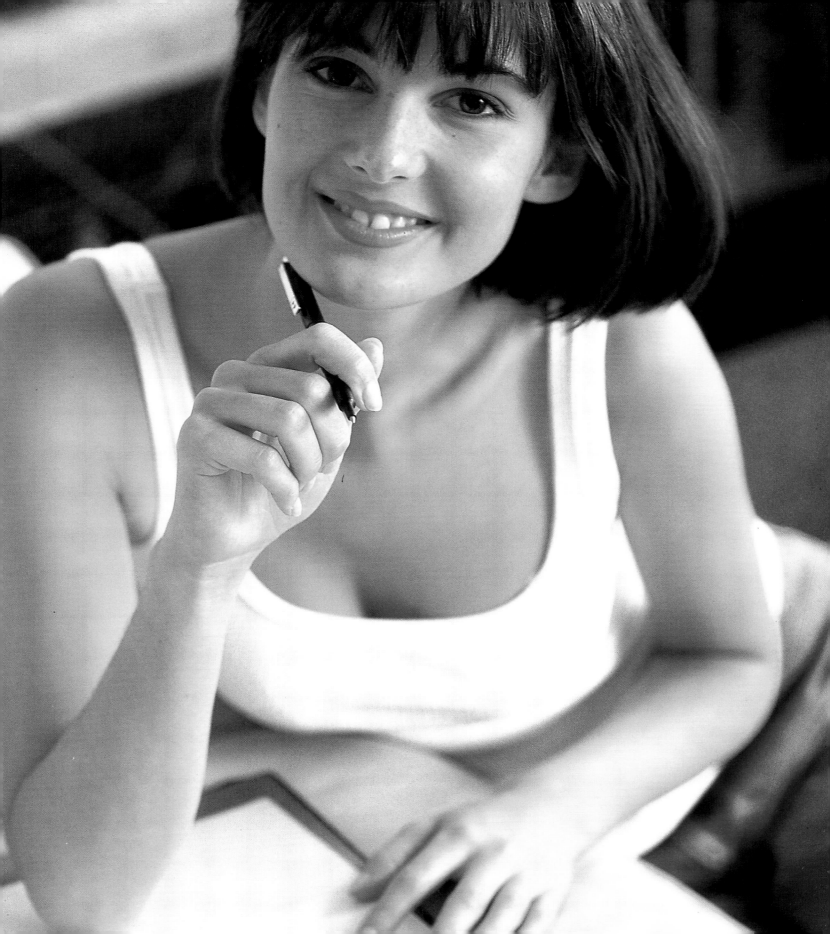

setting the scene

You do not need to spa alone. It is not imperative to banish your friends and family, and veto all stimuli such as the television and the telephone to benefit from your spa weekend. However, you may prefer to shield yourself from all distractions for a few days. There are no rules. Your spa is whatever you wish it to be.

preparing your spa

Creating the right environment is paramount, so be prepared to spend a little time getting your sanctuary ready:

● declutter – throw away junk, old books and magazines. Scrub the bath and change your bed linen.

● fill your home with fresh air – open windows to remove stale air.

● invest in green plants and fresh flowers – they bring life into an area and are energizing.

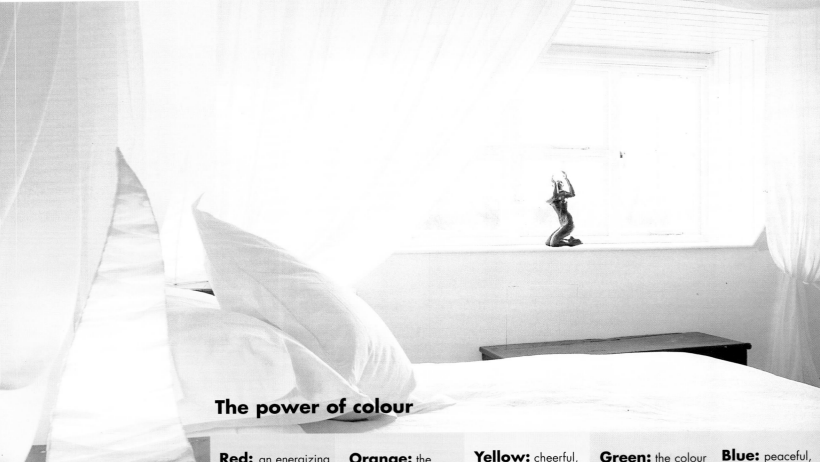

The power of colour

Red: an energizing colour that can increase your pulse, respiration and brain activity. Colour experts prescribe it for depression and tiredness.

Orange: the colour of fun and energy. It can lift the spirits and stimulate memory. Linked with sunshine and summer, it is a warm, revitalizing colour.

Yellow: cheerful, energetic, it can stimulate intellectual judgement. Good for boosting energy, but perhaps not in the bedroom as it may disturb sleep.

Green: the colour of balance, calm, and compassion. Green is the colour of life, and is said to help fatigue, insomnia, tension and anger.

Blue: peaceful, orderly, restful and soothing. Blue has been found to lower blood pressure and pulse rate and to reduce stress.

- lighting – reposition lamps to create soft lighting, buy candles for candlelit bathing, and maximize natural light for energy.
- be clever with colour – choose shades to complement your spa theme. White sheets, for example, promote sleep; red in the bedroom may over-stimulate you at night.
- drench your space in colour – drape coloured muslins or silks over doorways, scatter bright scarves and shawls over furniture; choose coloured fruits and cushions.

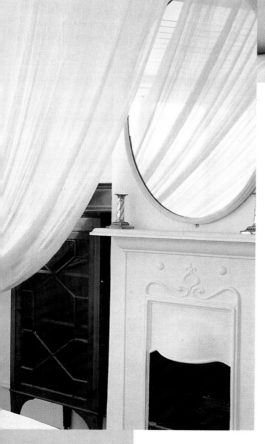

Violet: calming and soothing, violet and lilac shades create peace and tranquillity. It is often considered the most spiritual colour.

White: clean and calming, white suggests purity. It is a good antidote to sensory overload, and a good colour for meditation.

journey of the senses

A spa treatment should enliven each of your senses. It will only have far-reaching effects if it appeals to both your mental and physical state.

sights

Theories abound about the healing and energizing impact of our surroundings. This is hardly surprising when you consider that sight is our dominant sense, occupying three fifths of our conscious attention.

Colour therapists claim that the colours we place around us can affect our emotions. Psychologists have explained the reason for this. Colour affects the cellular structure of our bodies; different colours provoke different physiological responses. This physical reaction to colour results in turn in a psychological reaction – we react to every colour emotionally.

feng shui

According to the ancient – and increasingly popular – art of feng shui, you can maximize the flow of 'chi', or energy, in your surroundings by the way you decorate them and arrange your furniture, thereby making positive differences to your health, wealth, happiness and love life.

The basic tenets of feng shui – that clutter blocks energy, that living plants, natural fabrics and colours, good light, fresh air and harmonious surroundings enhance our wellbeing – make good sense. They are sound rules to follow when creating your own spa haven.

sounds

Visit any good spa retreat or reputable beauty salon, and you will be lulled into a state of relaxation by carefully chosen music or sound effects. Studies show that sound and music affect us emotionally, and can be a highly effective way of boosting our psychological and physical wellbeing. They are, as such, a vital ingredient in any home spa.

Sounds are made up of vibrations, which change the rhythm of our brainwaves and alter our heart rate or breathing patterns. For example, certain sound compilations have been found to relieve the symptoms of irritable bowel syndrome. Studies have shown that stress-reducing music has the power to reduce pain and anxiety in post-operative hospital patients.

Try to incorporate sound into your weekend spa. Think about your responses to different kinds of music and prepare a selection of tapes and CDs to play. If you need an energy boost, loud, upbeat music will raise your heart rate and shake you out of your lethargy. Gentle music, on the other hand, will slow your breathing, improve your concentration and soothe you.

Explore natural sounds – tapes of birdsong, bells, flowing water, the rainforest, or the ebb and flow of the sea can be simple but effective accompaniments to meditation.

scents

Using essential oils

When burned, essential oils are used neat. When used in massage, most of them – with the exception of lavender and tea tree (in small quantities) – should be diluted in a carrier, such as vegetable, almond or grapeseed oil. Not all essential oils are advisable for pregnant women or for those with certain medical conditions: always check the label for contraindications.

Oils to choose from

- Bergamot: antiseptic, antiviral, balancing, uplifting, controls anger and increases self-esteem
- Clary sage: warming and antiseptic, relaxing, soothes stress and anxiety
- Eucalyptus: antimicrobial agent, anti-fungal, purifying, cleansing, head clearing
- Frankincense: antiseptic, balancing, relaxing, tonic, soothes the emotions
- Geranium: astringent, stimulates the circulation, balances the emotions, refreshes the mind
- Grapefruit: astringent, refreshing, stimulating, detoxifying, emotionally cleansing, refreshing and revitalizing
- Juniper: antiseptic, detoxifying, stimulating, uplifting, refreshes tired muscles and aching limbs
- Lavender: comforting, restorative, soothing, dissolves tension
- Lemon: antiseptic, refreshing, stimulating, strong antibacterial agent
- Mandarin: tonic, relaxing, helps to destress
- Myrrh: antiseptic, relaxing, soothing, promotes tranquillity, eases tension and helps relax muscles
- Peppermint: cooling, anti-inflammatory, analgesic, invigorating, helps clear the head
- Roman chamomile: relaxing, antiseptic, helps to dissolve tension
- Rosemary: antiseptic, stimulating, invigorating, refreshing, antimicrobial agent, good for fatigue and general apathy
- Sweet marjoram: antiseptic, relaxing, warming, tonic, induces a relaxed state, soothing
- Tea tree: antimicrobial agent, immune-stimulant, morale booster, energizing
- Ylang ylang: soothing, comforting, balancing, evokes a harmonious state, sensual and self-indulgent

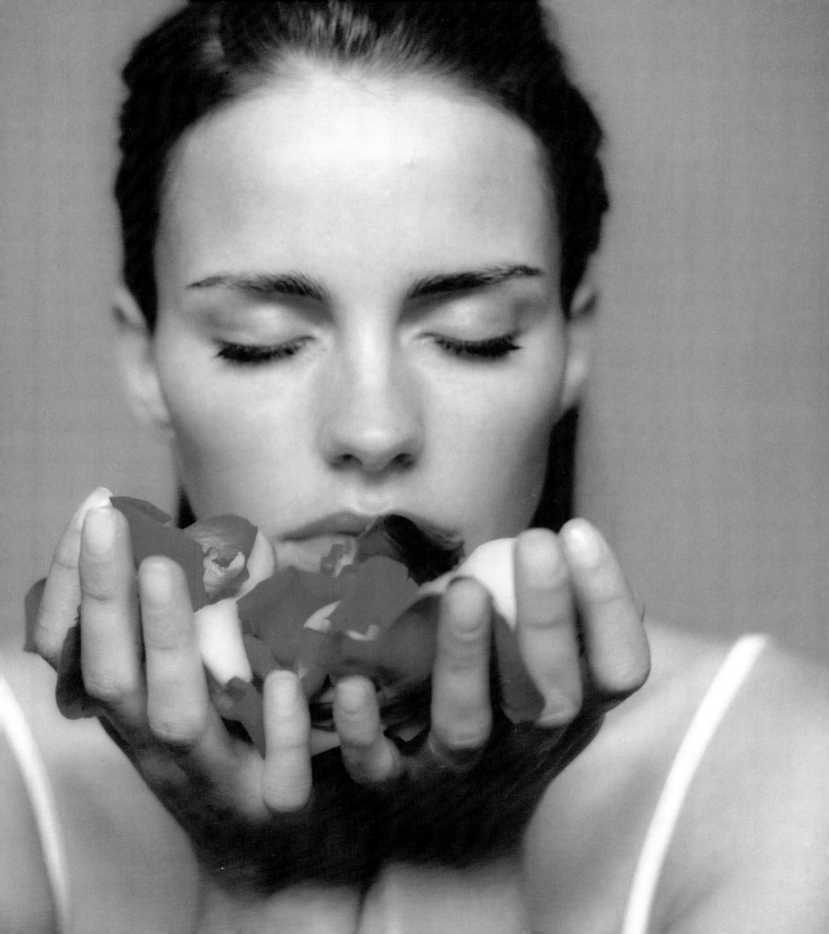

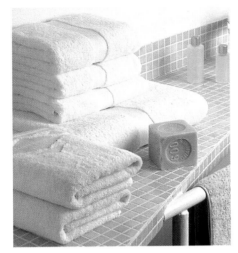

touch

You do not need a masseur to benefit from the healing power of touch. Self-massage can also stimulate the lymphatic system and skin, boost circulation and cellular renewal, and help speed up the elimination of toxic wastes.

Few treatments are more therapeutic and soothing than massage and manipulation therapies, and the amazing benefits of touch are well-documented. Patients who suffer from panic attacks and children with learning difficulties have apparently been helped by having their faces stroked with a fine paintbrush. It has also been medically proven that babies who are regularly massaged and touched develop better.

These days there are countless bathroom accessories – from loofahs to jacuzzi attachments – which can stimulate or soothe you. Invigorating water jets and jacuzzi baths can also boost the circulation and refresh the body.

Seek different sensations for your skin. Choose your lotions and potions, oils and powders carefully.

Surround yourself with a feast of fabrics such as crisp linen, warm fluffy towels, silk pyjamas, or the very softest cashmere.

tastes

Our sense of taste is often no ally in the battle against poor nutrition. Chips, chocolate and wine have each blighted many a good intention. According to the experts, pleasure from food is derived from much more than just taste – it has to do with appearance, smell and texture, too.

When preparing your spa fare, bear in mind that nutritionists maintain that a wide variety of flavours, colours and textures – as well as healthy but filling foods and occasional treats – will keep your taste buds satisfied for longer. Keep these health tips in mind:

● Spices, such as cinnamon or ginger, or salsa toppings can make healthy foods more exciting, yet add few calories and no fat.
● Brightly coloured fruits and vegetables, such as mangoes, papayas and bright green salads, increase the desirability of foods by making them look far more tempting. Food experts say that the more colourful a fruit or vegetable, the higher its nutritional value.
● Indulge yourself, but opt for low-fat or low-calorie substitutes, such as oven chips, skimmed-milk custard instead of cream and reduced-fat chocolate bars.
● Fill yourself up: fresh tomato soup, baked beans, potatoes and air-popped, plain popcorn are all high volume but low-fat foods.

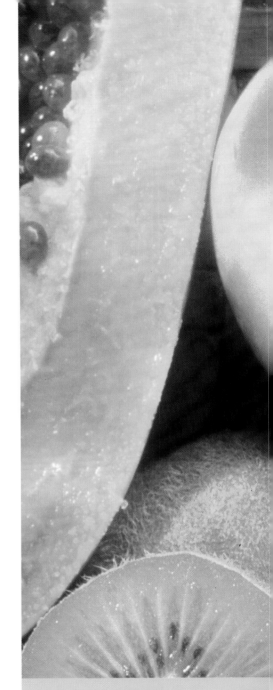

Shopping list

Here are a few accessories that can help you to take yourself in hand – and to turn your home into a spa.

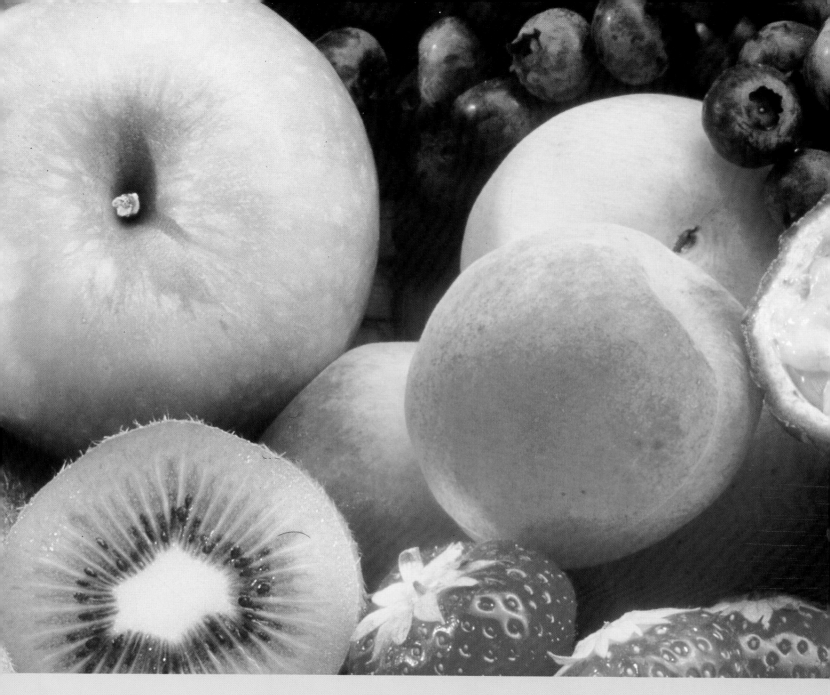

for the living room:
● flowers, throws, silk scarves, cushions, candles, CD or cassette player and disks, notebook, pencils, essential oil diffuser, incense sticks

for the bathroom:
● candles, fluffy towels, cotton wool, cotton buds, bath oils, body brush, bath salts, moisturizers, loofah

for the kitchen:
● fresh (preferably organic) fruits and vegetables, mineral water, carbohydrate-rich foods, such as wholegrains; live, natural yoghurt and organic honey;
for the Pampering Spa: chocolates and champagne (optional); see also individual spas for menu ideas and recipes

for the treatments:
● cleansers, moisturizers, exfoliators, body oils and lotions, mini manicure set, massage oils, mud or face masks, deep-conditioning hair treatment

for you:
● dressing gown, loose clothing for relaxation stretches, gym wear for exercise workout, cosy clothes

CHAPTER 2

cleansing Spa

eat, drink and think yourself purer

this is the spa to try if you have partied, indulged, lounged around and generally neglected your wellbeing in favour of sinful pleasures. Now is the time to purge yourself – but it won't be all sackcloth and ashes! Over this weekend you will eat fresh, nutritious foods, give your skin and body the attention they deserve and sweep the cobwebs from your head with some easy meditations and positive mindset exercises. By Monday, you won't know yourself.

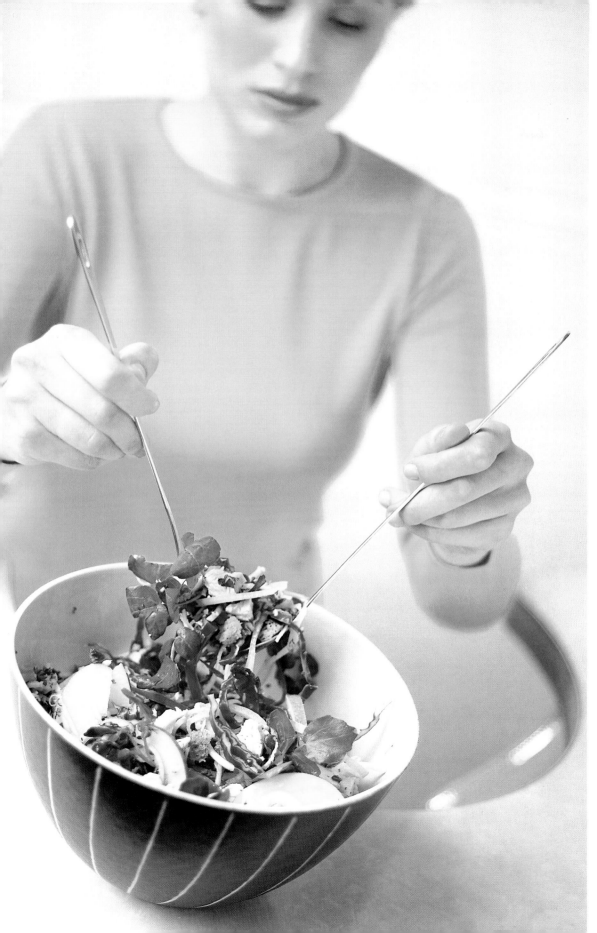

The cleansing eating programme

Don't worry. A radical detox is not on the agenda this weekend. Besides, that would only leave you feeling hungry and deprived; a better strategy is to try to give your system a light and delicious spring clean. So what to eat? Fresh, preferably organic fruit, vegetables and juices will provide a cleansing infusion of nutrients, while wholegrains (preferably not wheat-based) and nuts are good sources of soluble and insoluble fibre to stimulate healthy bowel action and leave you feeling light and refreshed.

foods that cleanse

For this weekend only, try to cut out red meat, chicken, fish, pulses, and wheat-based foods such as bread, pasta, and cereals. Instead, fill your plate with the following cleansing foods:

Fresh fruit

● Colourful fruits contain a broad range of body-protecting antioxidants, to mop up potentially harmful free radicals. Fruit is also rich in soluble fibre, which helps regulate appetite and blood-sugar levels.
● Pineapple contains bromelin, an enzyme that breaks down protein and speeds up digestion, so try to eat a portion each day.
● Papaya and avocado have excellent cleansing properties and are also good for body repair and rejuvenation.
● Grapes are good for cleansing the liver and kidneys.

Vegetables

● Choose a variety of colours, flavours and textures, and combine raw and cooked vegetables. As well as vitamins, minerals and antioxidants, vegetables supply insoluble fibre, which stimulates regular bowel function effectively.
● Beetroot is a powerful cleanser and a tonic for the liver.
● Combine celery and apple to remove excess carbon dioxide from the body.
● Raw asparagus cleanses the kidneys and bladder.

Plus:

● Nuts are a good source of protein, unsaturated oils and are full of powerful antioxidants such as vitamin E and selenium.
● Take a break from bread and cereals, and instead choose oats (for soluble fibre) and brown rice (for insoluble fibre).
● Live, natural yoghurt promotes growth of healthy bowel bacteria.
● Water is the most important tool in any cleansing programme to help flush out toxins, and also to help the body absorb the nutrients from foods. Food is like a sponge: if it is dry, you can't get the vitamins and minerals from it, but if it is saturated with water it swells and allows all the vitamins and minerals into your body. Aim to drink between 1.5 and 2 litres (2½ and 3½ pints) each day.

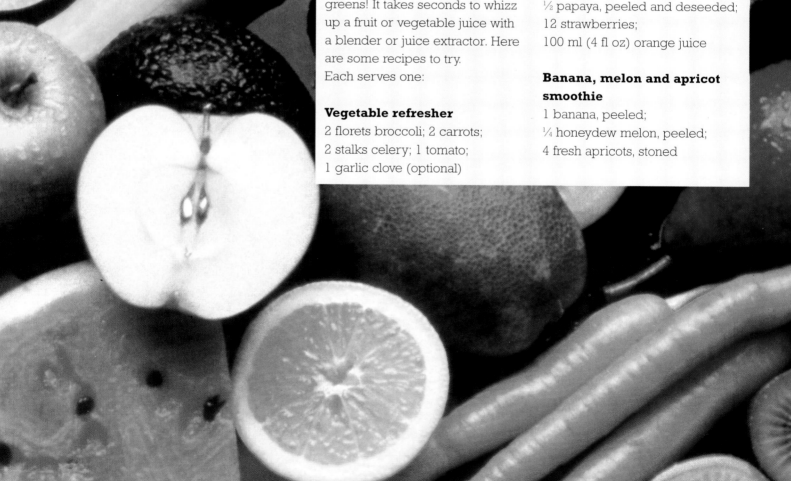

MEAL IDEAS FOR AN INNER CLEANSE

Saturday

Breakfast: fruit smoothie (soft fruit blended with yoghurt and honey to taste)

Lunch: Char-grilled Mediterranean vegetables with garlic and balsamic vinegar; mixed berries

Dinner: Stir-fried vegetables, hazelnuts and brown rice; strawberries and rhubarb poached in orange juice, basil and black pepper – topped with yoghurt

Snacks: Handful of nuts and dried fruit; juice; large slice of melon or pineapple; grapes; vegetable crudités with yoghurt and mint dip

Sunday

Breakfast: Sliced fresh fruit topped with oats, honey and yoghurt

Lunch: Pumpkin soup: homemade or supermarket fresh; fresh fruit

Dinner: Vegetable chilli with brown rice; lemon sorbet with fresh mango or papaya

Snacks: As for Saturday

Detox in a glass

Fruits and vegetables are packed with nutrients and are a staple of any cleansing food programme – but if you can't face munching all weekend, you can also drink your greens! It takes seconds to whizz up a fruit or vegetable juice with a blender or juice extractor. Here are some recipes to try. Each serves one:

Vegetable refresher

2 florets broccoli; 2 carrots; 2 stalks celery; 1 tomato; 1 garlic clove (optional)

Carrot and apple juice cooler

4 carrots; 1 apple

Papaya and strawberry cocktail

½ papaya, peeled and deseeded; 12 strawberries; 100 ml (4 fl oz) orange juice

Banana, melon and apricot smoothie

1 banana, peeled; ¼ honeydew melon, peeled; 4 fresh apricots, stoned

walk yourself fresher, fitter (and happier)

If you're embarking on this cleansing programme because you've put your body through the mill with parties and wild living, then vigorous exercise may not be an altogether inviting prospect. And yet physical activity is one of the best ways to help eliminate toxins, while also encouraging healthy and efficient digestion and raising your vitality levels.

Walking is the perfect activity for those in need of a gentle detox, or who want to take themselves in hand. With a walking workout, you can take it as fast or as slow as you wish, and – always a bonus – it is free. Plus, all you have to do to turn everyday walking into fitness walking is to lengthen your stride, quicken your pace, keep going and repeat regularly.

benefits of walking

Simply being out in the fresh air makes you feel healthier and more energetic, and it gives your mind a workout. It lets you appreciate your surroundings – smell the air, notice colours, listen to sounds – thereby taking the focus from your internal life. Walking can help put things into perspective.

According to research, brisk walking for 45 minutes four times a week can result in fat loss of over 8 kilos (18 lb) a year. In the long term, walking can reduce your risk of osteoporosis, strengthen your heart and lungs and reduce levels of LDL (harmful cholesterol) in the blood.

Walking can also improve your fitness as quickly as jogging, with less risk of injury. When two groups of women were studied over 13 weeks, (one on a walking programme, the other on a jogging programme) both were found to have gained the same health benefits, but the walkers had sustained fewer injuries.

The hardest thing to grasp when fitness walking is the pace. If you are used to walking at a gentle stroll, it isn't easy to know when you're walking hard enough to give your body a proper workout. Try using the 'perceived rate of exertion' scale on the top of the opposite page. It will help you to improve your fitness level gradually, in order to eliminate any risk of doing yourself harm.

Three ways to walk harder

● Carry light hand weights to exercise your upper body while you walk.
● For increased intensity and more variety, try interval training. Walk at a fast pace for say 400 m (360 yd), then slow down for the next 200 m (180 yd). Repeat as many times as is comfortable.
● Add hill-walking to your programme for a real challenge. It boosts aerobic capacity, heightens the cardiovascular workloads and trains your body to use oxygen more efficiently. Going uphill, lean into the hill, shorten your stride, try to keep your body perpendicular to the slope (leaning backwards can put strain on your back), and keep your knees soft to lessen the impact.

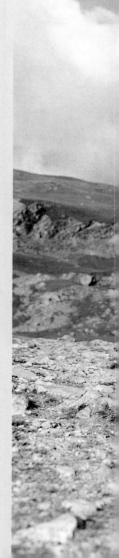

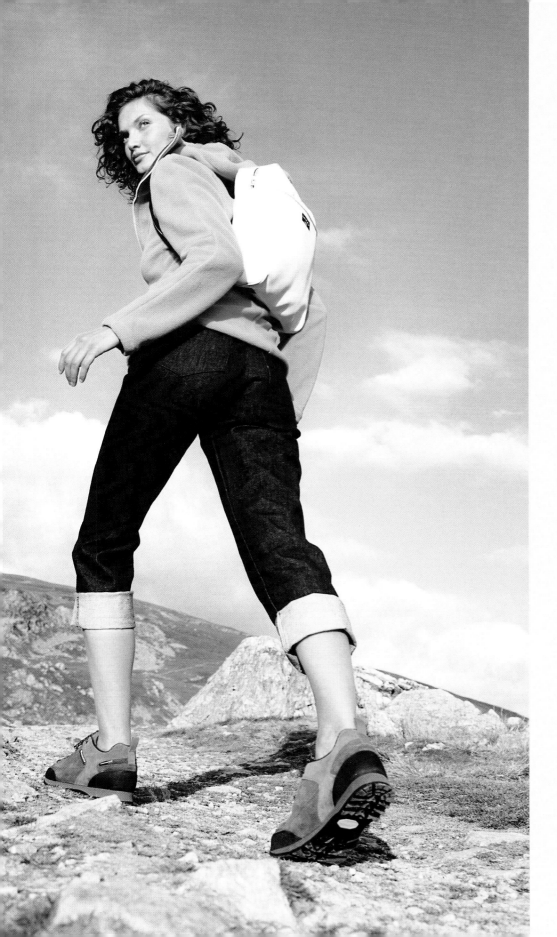

How fast?

Imagine a scale of 1 to 10 for effort: one is very comfortable, ten is extremely strenuous. Aim to work out at about six, so that your body temperature is raised and you feel warm but you are still able to carry out a conversation at the same time.

Walking tips

- Wear supportive shoes.
- Start with a warm up (see page 28).
- Maintain good posture: keep your shoulders back and your ribcage lifted. Strike forward with your heel and push off with your back foot.
- Gradually increase the length of your stride, but never overstretch. Keep your shoulders back and lift your ribs. Pull your abdominal muscles in and think tall. Look forward, not down.
- Listen to your body: increase the level when you no longer feel challenged: reduce the level when you feel tired. If you feel slightly breathless but comfortable, you are working at the right level.
- Don't increase speed at the expense of distance. Walking quickly for five minutes is not as beneficial as walking more slowly for ten.
- At the end of your walk, slow down gradually and repeat your stretching routine.

brush away the cobwebs

Over your Cleansing Spa weekend, aim for about four walks, of about 30 minutes each, minimum. If your Cleansing Spa finds you unfit and out of the habit of exercise, start slowly. Whatever your level of fitness, always spend three to four minutes warming up. Start with easy walking and some shoulder rolls, knee raises and side bends. Then work through these four key stretches.

1 *Hamstring Stretch*

Stand with one foot in front of the other. Transfer your weight to your back leg. Bending that leg, 'sit down' into the stretch. Support yourself on the thigh of the bent leg. Tip your pelvis, so the base of your spine tilts up. Keep your hips square. Hold for 8 to 10 seconds, feeling the stretch at the back of the thigh of the leg in front. Repeat with the other leg.

2 *Spine Stretch*

Stand with your feet slightly wider than hip-width apart, bend your knees and lower into a half-squatting position. Place your hands just above your knees to support you. Pull in your tummy and tuck your head and pelvis under to round your spine. Hold for 8 to 10 seconds, feeling the stretch down your back.

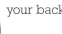
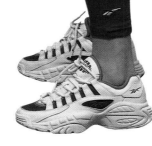

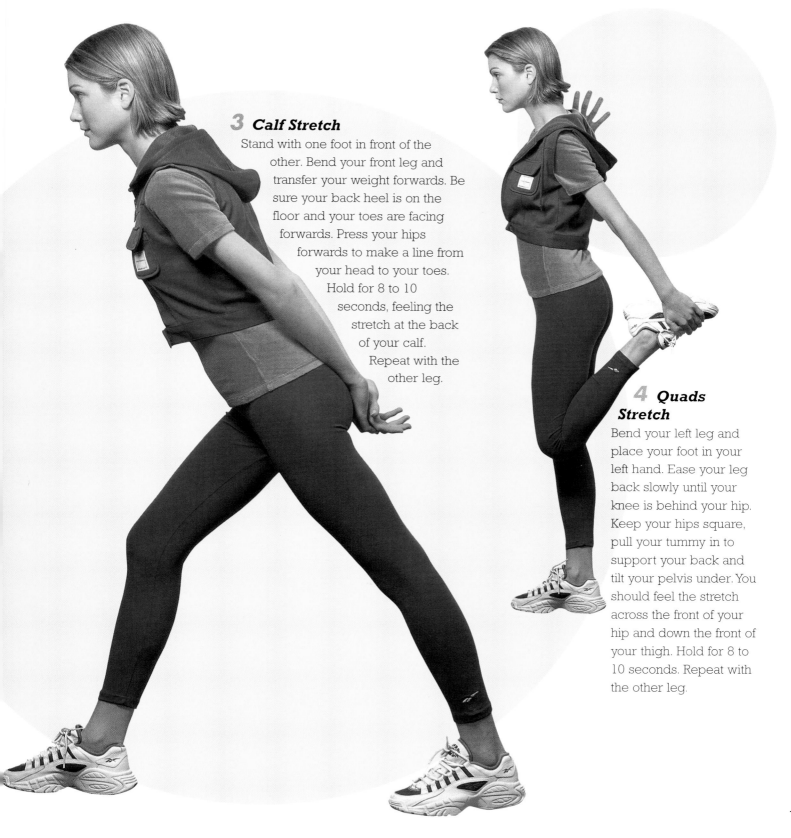

3 Calf Stretch

Stand with one foot in front of the other. Bend your front leg and transfer your weight forwards. Be sure your back heel is on the floor and your toes are facing forwards. Press your hips forwards to make a line from your head to your toes. Hold for 8 to 10 seconds, feeling the stretch at the back of your calf. Repeat with the other leg.

4 Quads Stretch

Bend your left leg and place your foot in your left hand. Ease your leg back slowly until your knee is behind your hip. Keep your hips square, pull your tummy in to support your back and tilt your pelvis under. You should feel the stretch across the front of your hip and down the front of your thigh. Hold for 8 to 10 seconds. Repeat with the other leg.

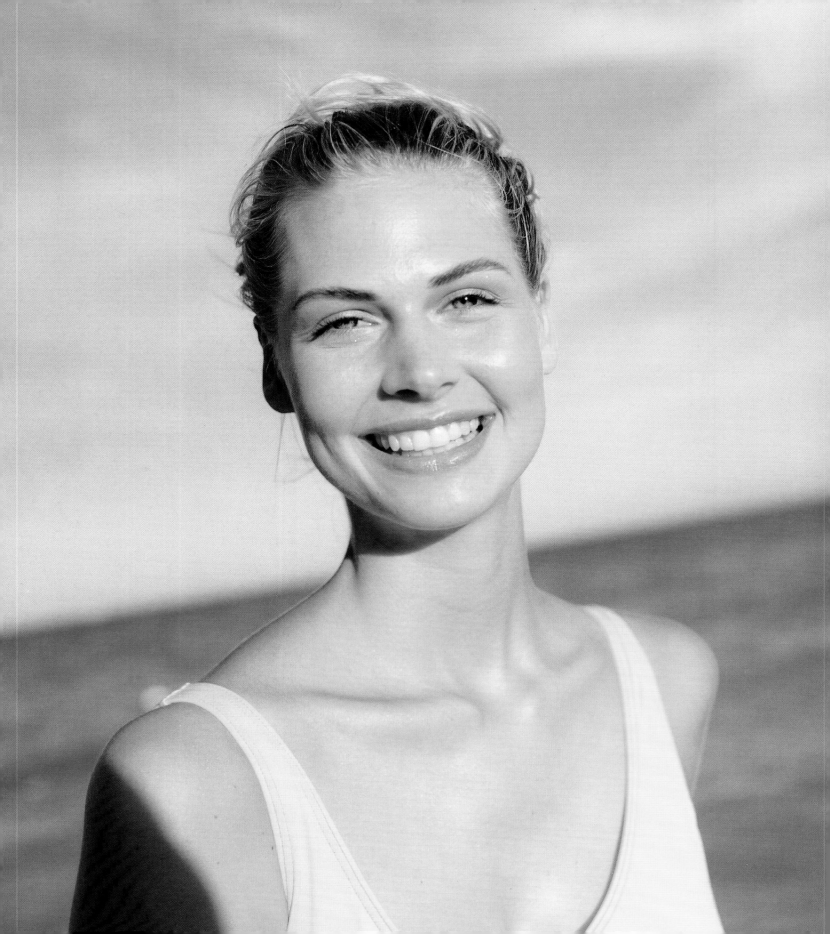

total spring-clean

If you've been committing all sorts of beauty sins (not removing eye make-up, skimping on moisturizers, that sort of thing), then now is the time for some thorough cleansing, salon style. The following routine should leave your skin deliciously clean. Try this once during your spa weekend (then try to incorporate it into your regular beauty routine).

face cleansing

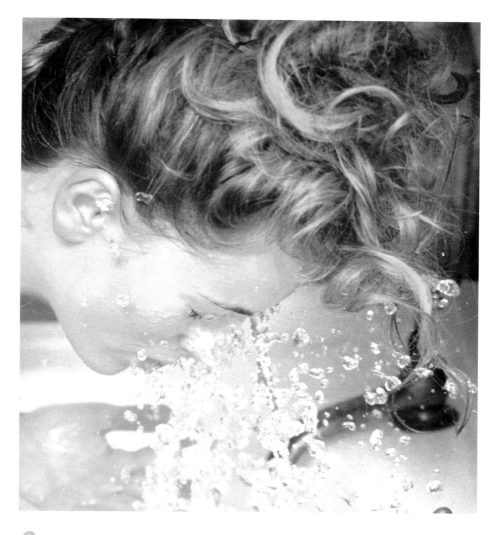

1 Use a gentle (petroleum-free) light lotion to dissolve waterproof make-up – to avoid causing dryness of the eye lashes or eye tissue. Avoid heavy-based creams which may cause puffiness and 'smarting' to the eyes. Always invest in a proper range of products; instead of using general facial cleansers use gentle, specially formulated eye products. Apply eye-make-up remover to damp, circular cotton wool pads and press gently over the eye area and lashes to effectively remove make-up. Work with light, gentle, inward movements, using the ring finger for least pressure. Avoid dragging the eye tissue as it is the most delicate area on the face. A good eye-make-up remover will also dissolve lipstick – it is particularly useful for dark colours which can sometimes stain your lips.

2 Cleanse your face using an appropriate product to suit your skin i.e. cream or milk for dry/sensitive skin, lotions for normal skins and gels or foaming cleansers, or non-oily lotions, for oily skins. It is not always necessary to apply to cotton wool or tissues as this can waste the product. Start at the base of your neck and work upwards in light, stroking movements. Work the product outwards and upwards on your face (avoiding the eye area). Remove any excess with a warm, wet, clean flannel or washcloth.

3 Exfoliation is a great way to remove dull surface cells and enliven your complexion. Rub in gently and rinse well.

4 Fill a bowl with warm water and a few drops of essential oil – such as lavender or eucalyptus. Put a towel over your head and inhale for five minutes to let the steam open the pores, making the removal of debris much easier. Now is also a good time for a spot of eyebrow tidying, as when the pores are open, hairs are easier to extract. (If you are prone to broken veins on your nose and cheeks, avoid this step.)

5 Apply a face mask. These days there is a vast choice of products on offer. Alternatively make your own (see the list of recipes on page 49).

6 Remove the mask with warm water. Pat your skin, then massage it with an aromatherapy facial oil. Always apply to damp skin, inhale deeply and apply lightly to the face, then massage it in.

7 Remove excess oil with a light toner, astringent or freshener. Avoid alcohol-based toners if you have very dry or sensitive skin, as they can be too drying. Toners freshen the skin and can temporarily make the pores appear smaller.

8 Apply eye gel working inwards, and avoiding the mobile part of the eyelid (which is thin and may become puffy).

9 Apply your moisturizer. Choose day creams, which protect your skin from pollution, UV rays and air conditioning. Dermatologists recommend using a minimum protection factor (SPF) of 15, even in winter.

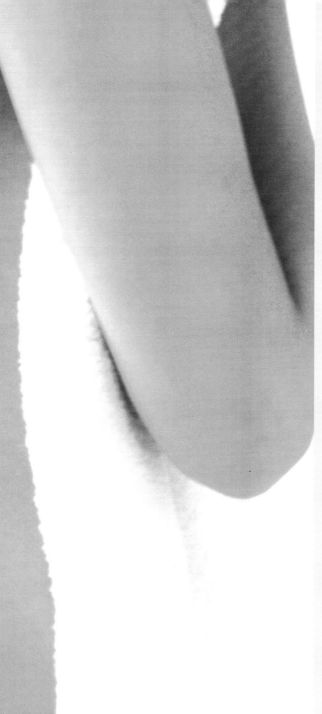

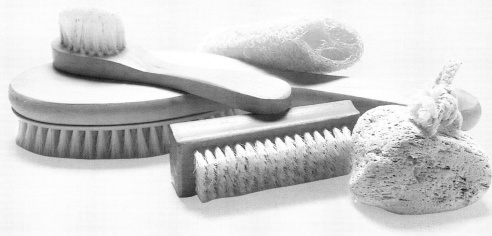

body cleansing

Skin brushing should preface any thorough body cleanse as it removes dead skin and aids absorption of the products. It boosts circulation and stimulates the lymph glands which are responsible for the elimination of toxins from the body. Try this once during the weekend, although it's a good idea to brush daily before a bath or shower generally. Use a big body brush, available from chemists or beauty counters. On dry skin, brush in long strokes towards the heart for five minutes.

Another great way to remove dead skin cells and revitalize a sluggish circulation is to exfoliate. Invest in one of the countless body scrub products on offer these days, or improvize with some rough sea salt and a loofah and scrub away. Buff gently in circles, paying particular attention to your knees, elbows and feet. Rinse off thoroughly. Give your skin a final blast with cold water.

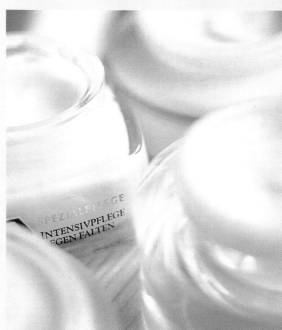

Don't forget that vital beauty rule: moisturize, moisturize, moisturize. Think delectable, fragranced creams, or rich, aromatherapy-based moisturizers.

cleanse your mind, declutter your life

this weekend spa is about cleansing yourself inside and out. That means clearing the clutter from your head too. Most of us are invaded by 'mind toxins' at some time or other; anger, frustration, negative thoughts and anxiety can all poison our self-esteem if allowed to fester.

There are all sorts of ways to clean out the detritus that threatens your wellbeing. During your spa weekend try some, or all, of the following techniques designed to banish the mental baggage and restore your self-confidence.

Start with your surroundings. Trawl through your cupboards, your wardrobe, even your address book, for possessions or people that are draining your space and energy. Think 'clean slate'. Start afresh. Right now.

Mind games

Detox your head with some easy meditations and exercises. Focus on the here and now. Past events, future plans, worries and woes can all distract us from the present. Stress experts advocate setting aside time each day to focus 100 percent on the moment, on the ordinary tasks we perform each day.

Find something absorbing to do whether it be streamlining your wardrobe, washing the dishes, arranging flowers, or eating a meal. The simpler the task, the better. Concentrate fully on the job in hand. Try not to daydream or let your thoughts wander. Don't allow yourself to worry, or to think about the future.

For example, use the 40 seconds or so it takes to wash your hands to focus on the sensations you feel – warmth, wetness, the slipperiness of the lather, rinsing and drying. The unbroken concentration will help push aside the anxieties that have been nagging you. Emerging from this period of undivided attention, however short, will leave you feeling remarkably refreshed.

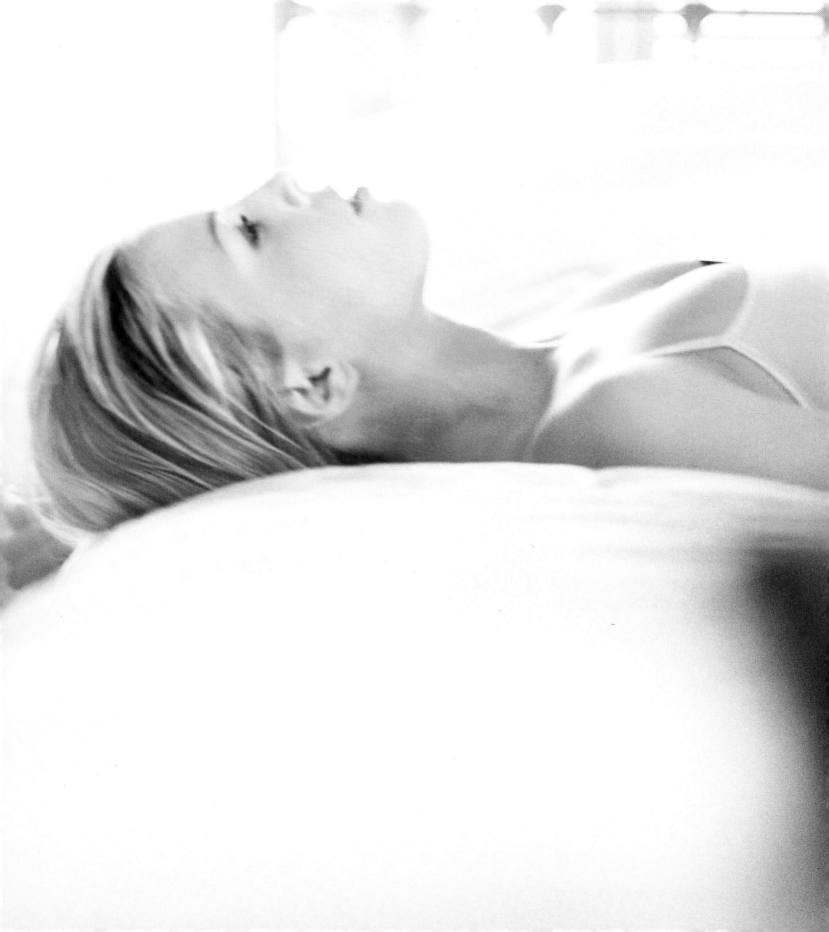

Think yourself purer

If your thinking is clear, life seems to go more smoothly. Meditating for 20 minutes a day is like taking a mental bath to wash away stress. Try the following exercise:

● If you have a radio alarm clock, set it to switch on quietly after 20 minutes. Alternatively, put a kitchen timer in a place, such as the next room, where you will hear it ring but where it won't be too loud.
● Pick a focus word with a peaceful, positive connotation, such as *calm*, *peace* or *love*.
● Sit quietly, close your eyes and consciously relax your muscles.
● Breathe slowly and naturally. Each time you breathe out, repeat your focus word silently.
● Be passive. Don't worry how well you are doing. When other thoughts come into your mind, dismiss them and keep repeating your focus word.
● Stay relaxed and passive for 20 minutes, continuing to repeat your focus word to yourself with each out breath.
● Let your thoughts return, sit still for another minute, then slowly stand up. Repeat the process twice a day over this weekend.

Get angry (on paper)

Anger, when repressed, can turn into resentment or depression. But writing down your anxieties and grievances is a powerful way to access your emotions, explore your psyche and set yourself on the path to healing. Writing about an unpleasant experience can help you to force it into a coherent story, and confront your more uncomfortable emotions. Bringing them out can also give you a sense of perspective.

This weekend get it out! Try writing a letter to anyone you feel angry with or resentful towards. (Or even write to life itself.) List his or her offences and explain how it made you feel and why. If you can, write 'I forgive you' at the bottom. Write as many letters as you wish. Imagine yourself purged of the pain or the anger. Then destroy the letters (just in case).

Create a happy, positive new leaf

Your imagination is a powerful tool that can help you to change bad habits and start afresh. Try this exercise: create a dull, grey picture on the 'mental screen' of your mind, of the thing you want to move away from (such as smoking, overeating or thinking pessimistic thoughts). Replace the picture with a big, bright image of what you want to move towards. In this way, you can make your fantasies work for you.

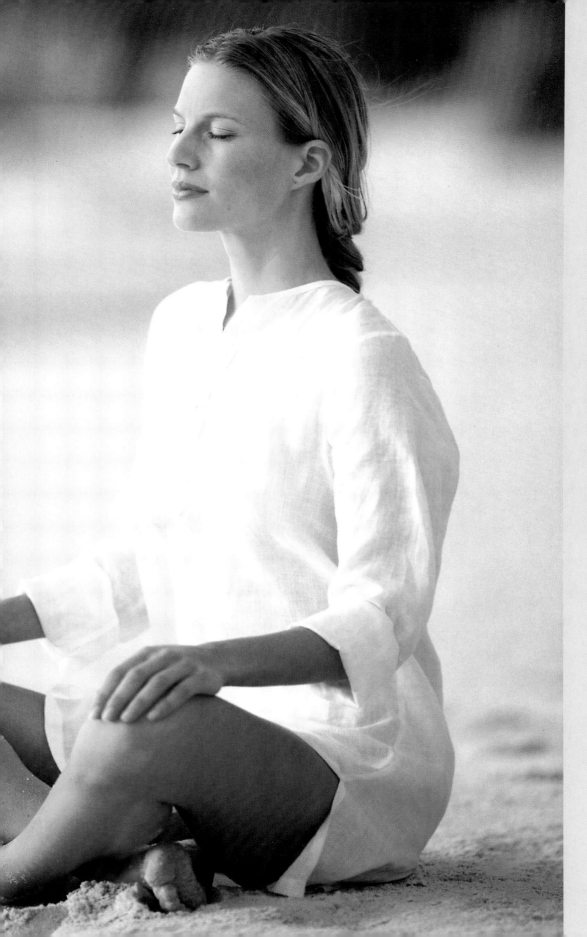

Visualize a detoxified you

Try this visualization exercise to detox your mind. Imagine your whole body suffused in cleansing and re-energizing white light that streams slowly through the top of your head. As it cascades down through you, imagine the toxins and negative thoughts being washed away.

better breathing

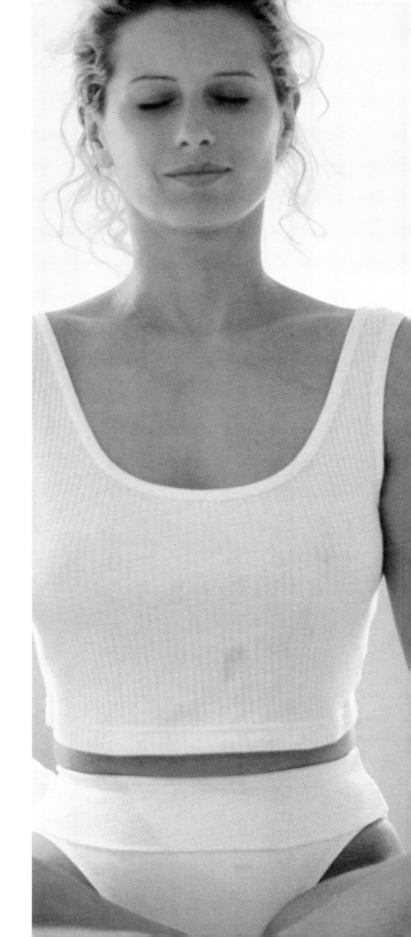

Think of breathing as giving your cells a mini spring-clean; every breath you take cleanses and nourishes your body. You may think of breathing as a simple, natural process. But many people do not breathe to their full potential.

Some people breathe too rapidly and too shallowly, often only using a fraction of their total lung capacity. This kind of breathing may be brought on by an asthma or panic attack, or, ironically, just by worrying too much about breathing. If your breathing is poor, your body is not getting enough oxygen, and in the short term, this can make you feel dizzy or lethargic and unwell.

How does it work?

Each time you breathe in, the oxygen molecules are absorbed from your lungs into your blood where they combine with haemoglobin (a pigment found in red blood cells) to produce oxyhaemoglobin, the compound that gives blood its bright red colour. Oxyhaemaglobin is then carried around your body in your bloodstream, delivering energy-providing oxygen to your body tissues and picking up carbon dioxide, the waste product of respiration, which is carried back to your lungs to be breathed out.

Exercise your lungs

Regular exercise is one way of getting more oxygen into your body. At rest, the average person breathes in about 0.5 litres (¾ pint) of air with every breath. During heavy exercise, when your muscle cells need more energy, your air intake can increase to 4.5 litres (7 pints) per breath. By getting your breathing muscles into better shape, you're making sure that they will work more effectively for you.

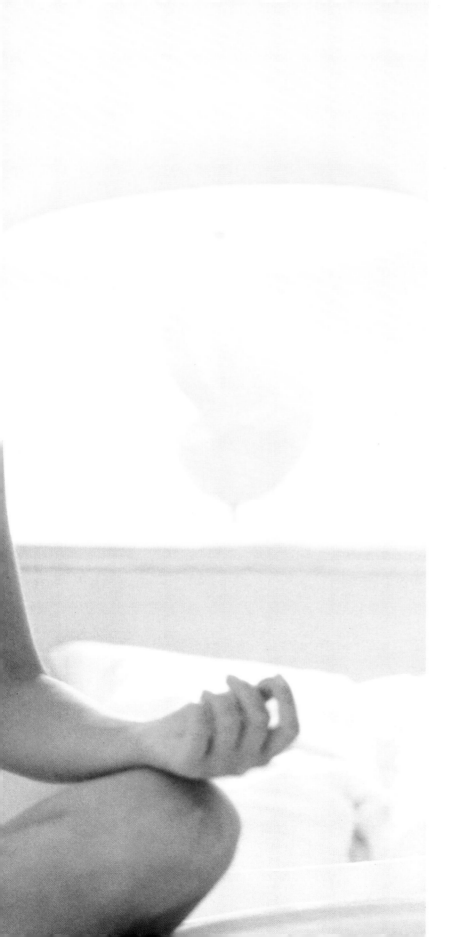

Learn to breathe again

During your spa weekend, set aside five or ten minutes each day to practise breathing from the abdomen, not from the chest. As you inhale, feel the breath entering your body through your nostrils, and let your stomach swell. Count slowly as you breathe in and out – take as long to exhale as you do to inhale. Feel the air you expel float away.

Exercise

Try the following yoga technique. Do this whenever you need a calm moment.

1 Sit cross legged on the floor, with the thumb and index finger of each hand together and your hands resting palm up on your knees. Lengthen your spine, keeping your shoulders down and relaxed.

2 Bend the three middle fingers of your right hand into the palm, allowing your thumb and little finger to stick up. Block your right nostril with your left little finger and breathing deeply through your left nostril, close your eyes, relax and inhale for five seconds. Exhale for five seconds. Repeat ten times.

3 Release your little finger from your right nostril and block your left nostril with your thumb. Close your eyes, relax and inhale for five seconds. Exhale for five seconds. Repeat ten times.

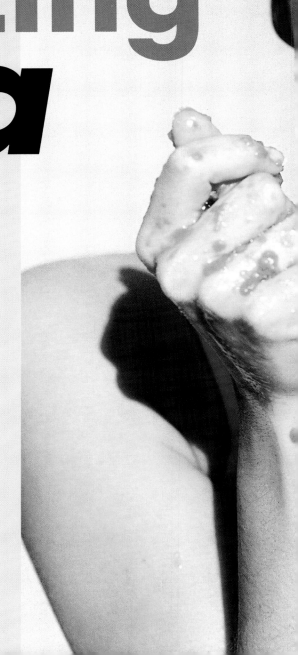

CHAPTER 3

energizing Spa

freshen up inside and out

feeling tired and lacklustre? You won't be for long. By eating properly, taking gentle, energy-boosting exercise and focusing on your skin and hair you can restore your glow and vitality in one weekend – without necessarily needing more sleep.

Eating for energy

Invigorated and revitalized are what you want to be this weekend. That means eating the right mix of carbohydrates, plus foods containing the maximum energy-releasing micronutrients (B vitamins, magnesium and iron). Follow these eating guidelines, and feel your vitality soar.

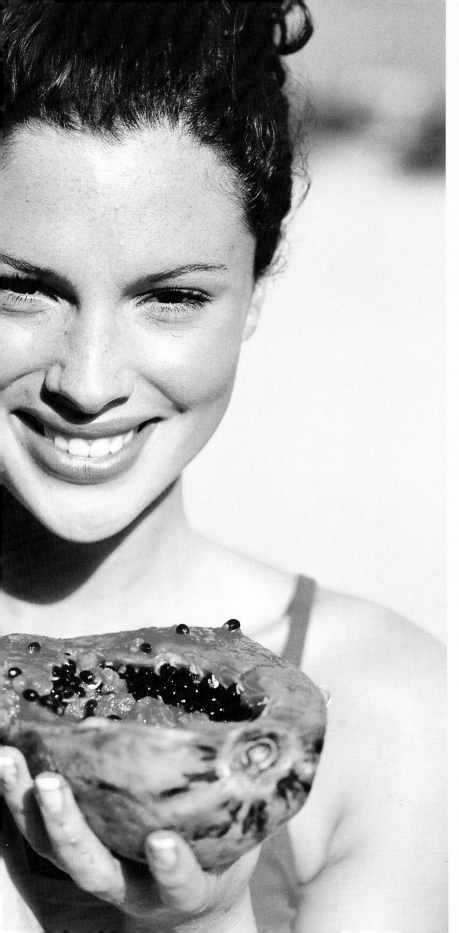

BEST FOODS FOR ENERGY

Your guide to carbohydrates

The glycaemic index (GI) is a measure of how quickly a food increases blood-glucose levels (BGLs). Low-GI foods are slowly digested and absorbed, gradually increasing your BGLs, to give a sustained energy release. High-GI foods are quickly absorbed and give a rapid, but less sustained, energy boost.

Low GI foods: Pulses, oats, bran based cereals, heavy-grain breads, pasta, basmati rice, fruit loaf, non-tropical fruit and juices, pitta bread, milk, yoghurt.

High GI foods: White and wholemeal bread, potatoes, rice, tropical fruits, root vegetables, refined cereals, biscuits, confectionery, soft drinks.

TO GET MAXIMUM ENERGY, eat a low-GI, light meal approximately two hours before you exercise. After your exercise session, choose high-GI foods, which refuel your muscles' glycogen (carbohydrate) stores.

Energy-Releasing Micronutrient Foods

MAGNESIUM SOURCES:
fish, green vegetables, nuts, wholegrain breads and cereals, potatoes

B VITAMIN AND IRON SOURCES:
red meat, oily fish, fortified breakfast cereals, wholegrain breads, green vegetables

MEAL IDEAS FOR MAXIMUM ENERGY

Saturday	Sunday
Breakfast: Porridge with diced, dried apricots and semi-skimmed milk	**Breakfast:** Muesli topped with grated apple and semi-skimmed milk
Lunch: Pitta bread filled with chicken and mixed green leaves, fruit yoghurt	**Lunch:** Bean and tuna salad, green salad and granary roll; cherries
Dinner: Pasta with salmon and spinach, baked apple	**Dinner:** Stir-fried chicken or tofu, spices and Asian greens with noodles; fruit compote (simmer favourite dried fruits and half a cinnamon stick in orange juice) topped with fromage frais
Snacks: High GI – cornflakes, jacket potato, banana, watermelon, jelly beans	**Snacks:** As for Saturday
Low GI – fruit yoghurt, fruit loaf, apple, orange, pear, grapes, beans on toast	

exercise for energy

the last thing you want to do when you feel exhausted and lacking in energy is to exercise, right? And yet it is just what you need to feel alert and revitalized – and that goes for any type of exercise from a walk on a beach or a step class, to just dancing around your sitting room.

It's true that there are times when flopping down on the sofa or having a sleep will do you more good than taking exercise. But it is important to listen to your body. Ask yourself if moving that worn-out body could actually boost your energy levels. Usually, the answer is yes.

Exercise is a great stressbuster because it distracts you from the day's events, but also because it switches your focus from your brain to your body. Exercise can also help dissipate the tension and fatigue you feel after a stressful day, tire you out physically and help you sleep better.

The more you exercise, the more efficient your body becomes at storing glycogen (carbohydrate) and at using fat as an energy source. As your heart and lungs become stronger, with every beat your heart pumps more blood, and therefore oxygen, around your body – and daily activities become less tiring.

Which exercise works?

The type of exercise you like doing most works best, so choose something enjoyable during your energizing weekend.

● Aerobic exercise is most likely to energize you, because it releases feel-good hormones called endorphins. It also has a long-term effect on your cardiovascular efficiency and boosts your metabolic rate. Try dancing, rollerblading, walking or playing a sport – choose any activity that you enjoy and which you do not see as a chore.

● You need to work relatively hard to experience what is known as 'runner's high'. A 20-minute jog won't do it, but working out at a high intensity for at least half an hour will. Don't overdo it, and if you have not exercised for some time, start with short sessions. In the long term, aim to fit three to five exercise sessions – of 30 to 60 minutes – into your week.

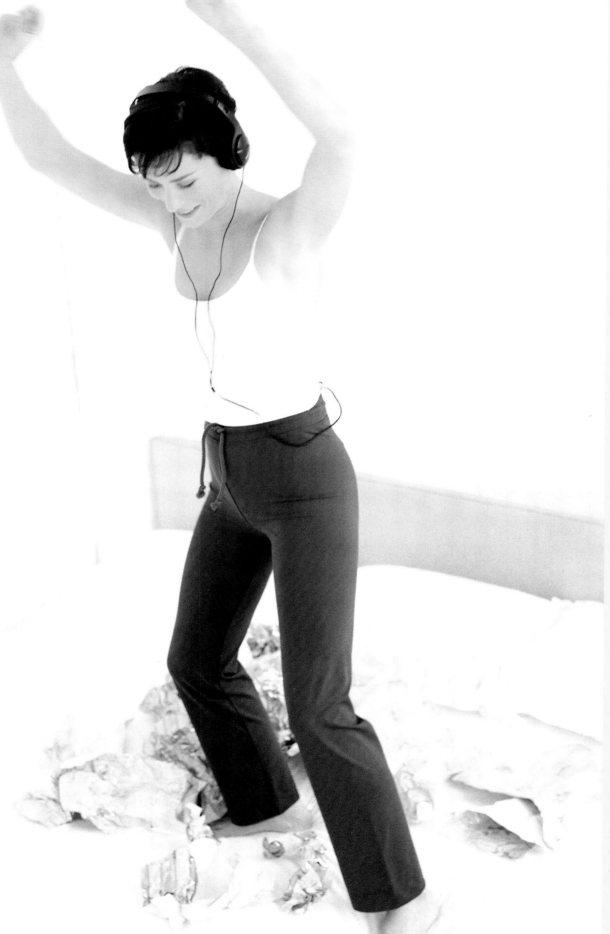

RELEASE THE TENSION

Aerobic exercise is only one part of the fitness picture. Stretching is another important way of releasing muscular tension and stress. Yoga and t'ai chi are very effective as they help you to wind down, and also make you focus more on breathing deeply. This will increase your energy level and boost the amount of oxygen reaching your brain and muscles (see page 56 for t'ai chi moves designed to impart energy).

This weekend, aim for between 30 and 60 minutes of aerobic activity (walking, dancing, etc.), either in one session, or divided into two or three sessions. Always stretch before and after your workout. Devise your own workout or try the energizing workout on pages 44 to 47.

move it, shake it

If you want a new way to exercise, without having to pull on your trainers and drag yourself down to the gym, try NIA (which stands for Non-Impact Aerobics or Neuromuscular Integrative Action). All you need is floorspace, some music and comfortable clothes. Oh, and a bit of rhythm.

NIA is a mind-body-spirit technique that integrates aerobic conditioning, balance and flexibility. Although high in energy, it is both safe and adaptable to people of virtually any fitness level. It is a combination of Eastern and Western movements incorporating

taekwondo, t'ai chi, yoga, Alexander Technique, rolfing, jazz and dance – set to music. Unlike traditional classes, there are no set structures or movements to follow; this is all about allowing your imagination to move your body, and you can do it in the comfort and privacy of your own home. The workout can involve dancing like a ballerina one minute, shouting and stamping your feet like a child the next.

NIA not only offers aerobic conditioning, it enhances neuromuscular co-ordination and can give you the kind of fitness you can use in day-to-day activities. It's

also easy to do, fun, and leaves you feeling refreshed and energized, making it an ideal workout to fit into your energizing spa weekend.

Ideally, this workout should be done three times a week. (One day this weekend could be your first session.) The workout should take about half an hour, with each exercise lasting about four minutes. Try to make the movements slow and flowing but there are no hard and fast rules, this is about self-expression. Put on your favourite music – or try Annie Lennox's *Medusa* or *Shepherd Moons* by Enya in the background. Get moving and enjoy it.

the energizing workout

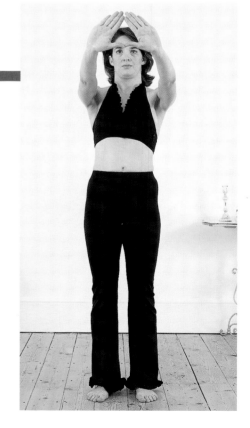

The Triad

1 Stand with your feet hip-width apart and your knees slightly bent.

2 Stretch your arms out, touching your thumbs and forefingers together to make a triangular shape in front of your face. Look through the triangle and breathe. Relax your shoulders. Think GRACE: Grounded, Relaxed, Aware, Centred, Energetic.

3 Concentrate on feeling the ground beneath your feet and, as you look through the triangle, focus on your intentions for the workout. Picture yourself as an athlete preparing for an event.

The Robin Hood

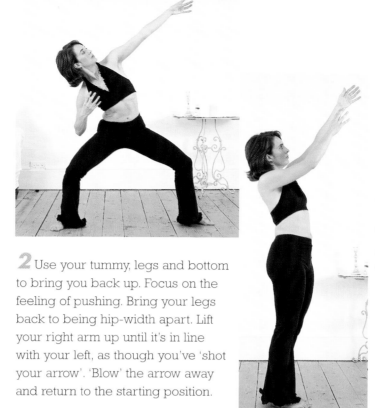

1 Stand with your feet hip-width apart. Take one step back and to the side, so that your legs are wide apart, with your feet pointing out and your knees over your feet. Raise your left arm, so your fingers are pointing to the point where the wall meets the ceiling. Keeping your pelvis stable, bend your knees, inhale and lean back. Look along your extended arm and bend your other arm as if you're holding onto a bow (see picture). Point your outstretched fingers where your 'arrow' is to go and invite the feeling of open space between your ribs and left hip.

2 Use your tummy, legs and bottom to bring you back up. Focus on the feeling of pushing. Bring your legs back to being hip-width apart. Lift your right arm up until it's in line with your left, as though you've 'shot your arrow'. 'Blow' the arrow away and return to the starting position.

3 Repeat the whole series of movements eight times on each side. Reduce the repetitions to four times on each side, then twice on each side, then once each side.

The Cape

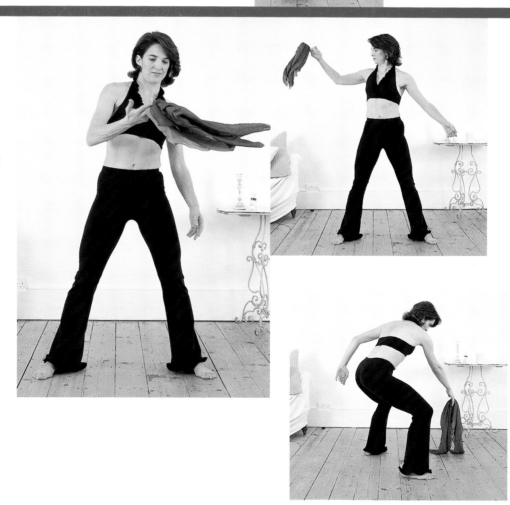

1 Stand with your feet wide apart. Bring your right hand across your body and over to the left in a sweeping, circular motion, as if you are wearing a cape and wrapping it over your shoulder. If you like, use a piece of clothing to help you.

2 Now repeat the same movement with your left hand.

3 Repeat these two moves, but now start to bend your knees deeply. As you sweep to the left with your right hand, turn your right foot inwards; as you sweep to the right, turn your left foot in. As you 'sweep and sink', exhale. As you rise up, breathe in and smell the air, filling yourself with new energy. Continue for three minutes.

the workout continued

The Angel

1 Stand with your feet hip-width apart. Raise your arms up and at the same time, step forward onto your left foot, roll up onto the ball of that foot and raise your right leg behind you off the floor. While you're up there, imagine you are an angel with wings.

2 Return to the starting position. Move both hands out to the side, parallel to the floor. Imagine you have laser beams coming out of your fingertips, lighting up your room. Say 'Huh!', or, if you've had a bad day, 'No!', or 'Yes!'

3 Repeat eight times on each side. Reduce the repetitions to four times on each side, then twice on each side, then once on each side.

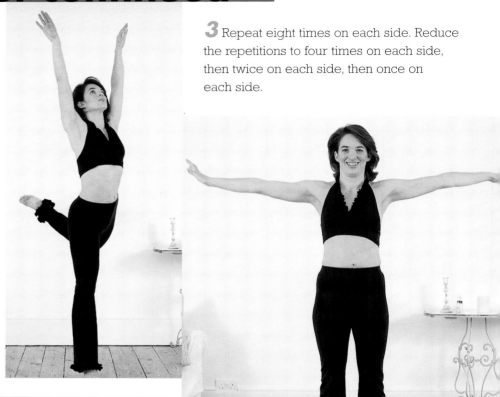

The Wave

1 Stand with your feet hip-width apart and your knees soft. Raise your arms above your head and reach up tall.

2 Then bend your knees and sink downwards, lowering your arms at the same time. Inhale as you rise up and exhale as you sink down.

3 Repeat eight times. As you move, visualize yourself moving with the ocean. Allow your body to flow and the waves to be continuous. You are a wave flowing from sea to sky.

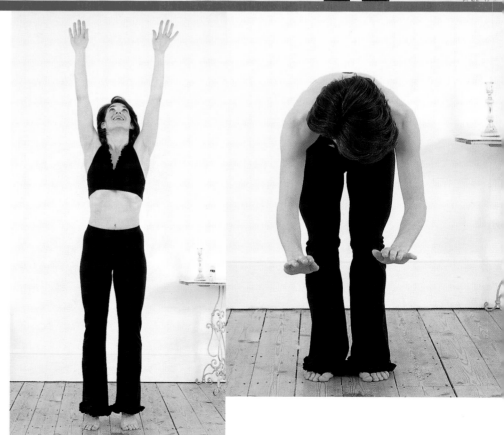

The Bubble

1 Cool down and stretch by imagining you are inside a huge bubble. Use any and every part of your body to press all sides of the bubble outwards. Really focus on the feeling of reaching and stretching. Become aware of the various parts of your body that need to be stretched more than others. Think of all your moves as cat-like.

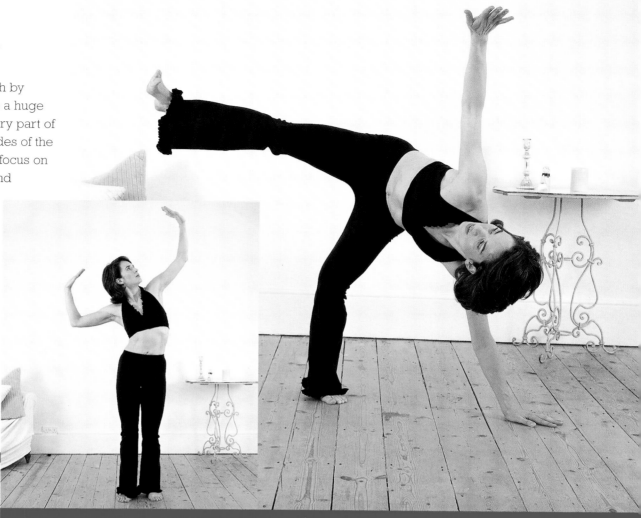

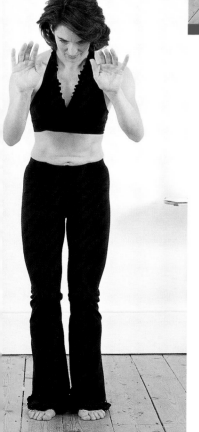

The Triad

1 Return to the first move of the workout. Recognize that the workout is coming to an end and remember to think GRACE.

2 Looking through your first triangle, take three slow breaths; the first inhalation signifies the past; the second inhalation the present, and the third inhalation the future. As you take the third breath, take two steps forward, walk 'through' your triangle and into the future.

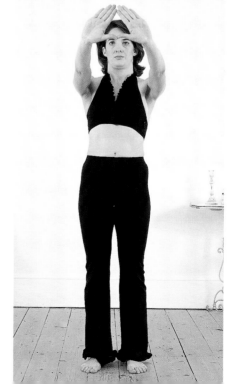

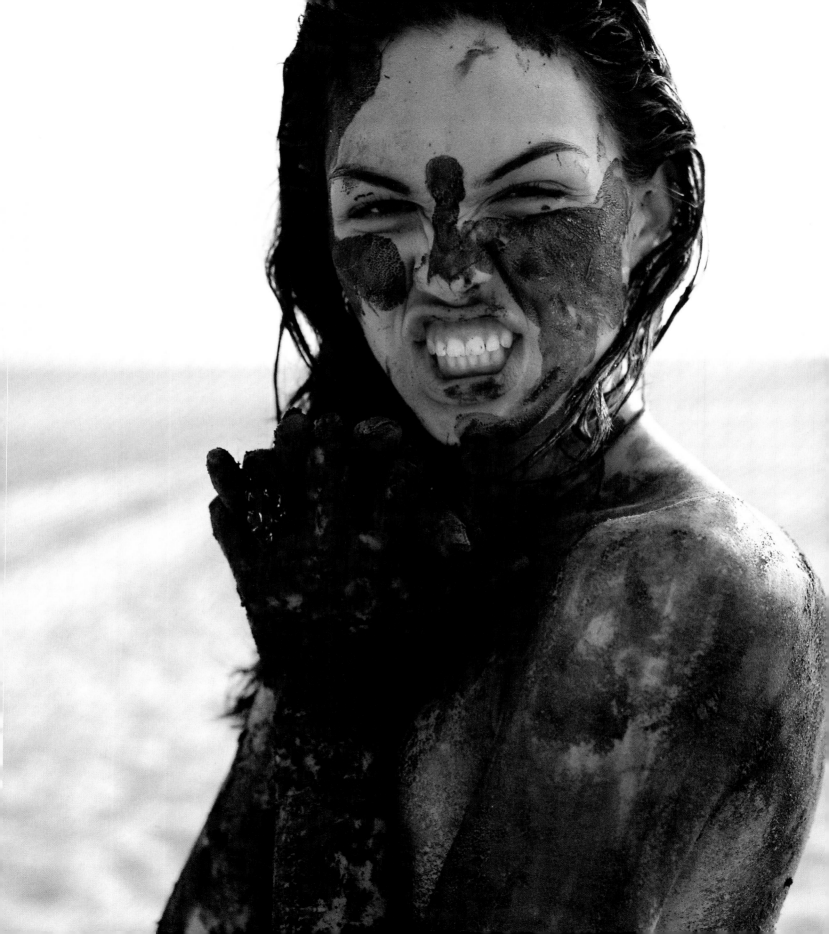

scrub your way to sexy skin

What is getting between you and radiant, glowing skin? Lack of sleep or poor circulation, or a haphazard diet? Or lots of nasty, dead cells? Or all of the above? The food guidelines and the exercise ideas should certainly help in the pursuit of a radiant complexion, as will a thorough facial, (as outlined in the Cleansing Spa on pages 31 to 32).

top scrubbers

Don't skimp on the exfoliation/mask stage of your routine because just the application and removal of masks and scrubs brightens the complexion and gives you immediate results. It works by removing surface cells leaving flatter, smoother skin that glows because it reflects light better. Detoxifying mud or algae masks are good for buffing up body and face, and will bring back memories of deliciously disgusting childhood days playing with mud pies!

Homemade scrubs

As if there weren't countless products on the shelves to choose from, your very own kitchen is a beauty parlour waiting to happen. Try whipping up your own simple recipes for a variety of masks and scrubs. Always make sure that your face is cleansed before applying facial masks:

Gentle exfoliator
(for sensitive skin)
2 heaped teaspoons fine oatmeal
2 teaspoons double cream
Combine the ingredients and rub into the skin lightly, using the balls of your fingers and avoiding the eyes, then rinse off.

Oatmeal scrub
2 tablespoons finely ground oatmeal
1 tablespoon almond oil
Combine and rub into the skin avoiding the eyes, then rinse off. (This scrub is also suitable for all-over body use.)

Cleansing mask
2 heaped teaspoons flour
1 teaspoon water
1 teaspoon honey
Mix together to a sticky consistency. Apply to affected areas, avoiding the eyes. Leave for five to seven minutes, then rinse off.

Moisturizing mask
1 egg
1 tablespoon sunflower/olive oil
Blend the egg and the oil together and smooth over your face, avoiding the eyes. Leave for 10 to 15 minutes, then rinse off.

Polenta and yoghurt scrub
1 tablespoon ground cornmeal (polenta)
2 tablespoons natural yoghurt
For invigorated, glowing skin. Mix into a paste and gently rub into the skin in small circular movements, starting at the chin and working up to the cheeks and forehead, avoiding the eyes, then rinse off.

Vitamin E-rich avocado mask
1 avocado
A soothing, moisturizing natural treatment. Mash the avocado flesh into a soft paste and apply to the face, avoiding the eyes, massaging it in with the avocado stone. Wash off with warm water.

Body-glow scrub
1 cup runny honey
½ cup sesame seeds
sprinkling of dried herbs, such as lavender leaf or mint
Mix together into a sticky paste and smooth over your body in slow circular movements. Shower off with warm water.

Follow your scrub/mask routine with the rest of the facial treatment steps as prescribed on pages 31-32.

the secrets of glossy hair

Is your hair behaving badly? The state of your hair can reflect your health and inner wellbeing, which can, in turn, affect your mood and confidence. This weekend is the time to give your hair the attention it so richly deserves.

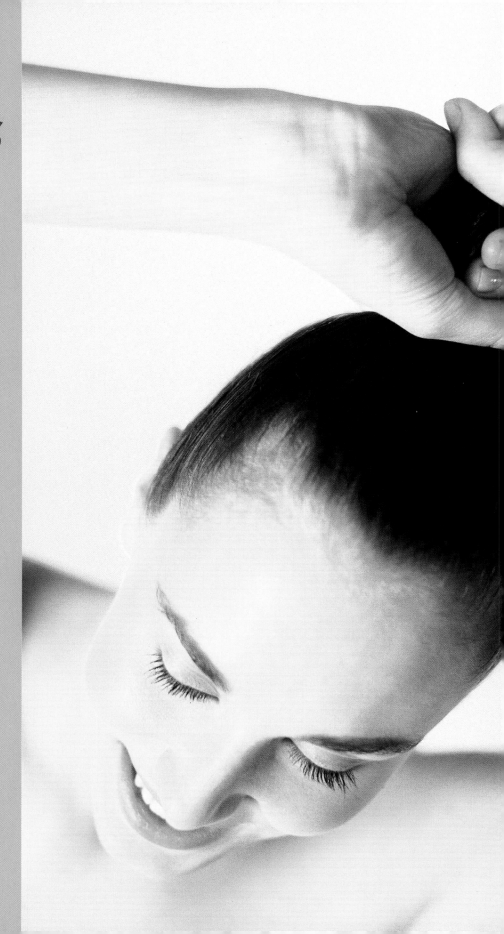

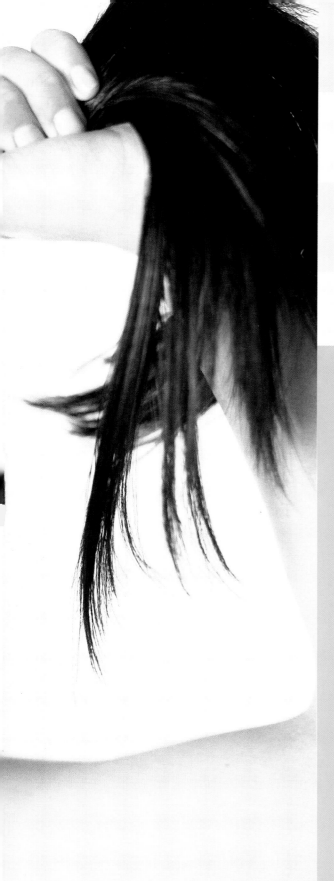

how healthy is your hair?

1 Hold a strand of hair between two pairs of tweezers, about 7.5 cm (3 in) apart and pull. Healthy hair should stretch 30 percent more – about 2.5 cm (1 in) – before it breaks. If it breaks sooner, it may have lost elasticity due to poor diet or chemical/styling damage.

2 Run your fingers through your hair and feel your scalp. If it feels tight (with little movement of the skin), your circulation may be poor. If it feels spongy, your scalp may be suffering from inflammation or a build-up of toxins, and will benefit from a scalp massage.

3 If your hair feels rough after shampooing (before conditioning), it may be because your shampoo is too harsh. Try using one with conditioning oils or one for combination hair.

There's no substitute for a good trim when your hair needs it, but if it's shine and bounce you're after, try the following treatments, designed to rein in even the most unruly locks.

conditioning oil

Condition your hair with conditioning oil (available in block form from most supermarkets). Warm 4 to 5 tablespoons of the oil until it liquefies and then, using cotton wool, apply it to every inch of your scalp. Leave it on overnight – protect your pillow with a towel. Wash the oil out of your hair the next morning.

scalp massage

Concentrate on cleansing your scalp rather than your hair, using a conditioning shampoo that contains oils such as jojoba or sweet almond oil. Even greasy hair benefits from these oils, as they trick hair into believing it is producing the oils itself, thereby regulating further production. When you are shampooing, focus on massaging your scalp with your palms and fingertips, to relax the skin, encourage blood circulation and help increase cell renewal.

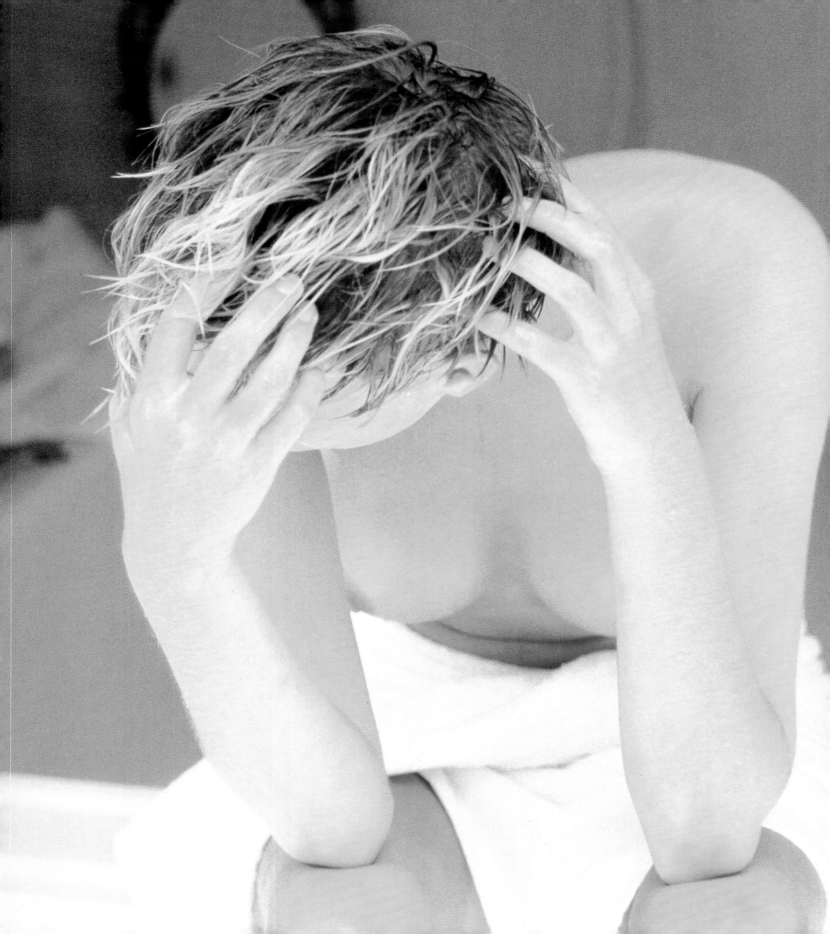

the ultimate shampoo

Damaged hair looks dull because the cuticles are disturbed or weakened. When the cuticles lie flat, your hair looks shiny and it's also better protected from further damage. This weekend, set aside half an hour for a thorough shampooing. Here's how:

1 Shampoo gently, working down the shafts of the hair in line with the cuticles, in even sections. Don't rinse your hair in bath water, as this contains alkaline soap residues that leave dulling deposits on the hair.

2 Rinse with cold water from a jug, or finish with a cold blast from the shower to tighten the cuticles. Or rinse with the juice of a lemon (or a capful of vinegar) diluted in a litre (2 pints) of cold water – the acid tightens the cuticles. Condition and rinse again.

3 Avoid towel drying, as this can tangle the hair and roughen the cuticles. Dry your hair on the coldest setting of your hairdryer – overdrying is the biggest hair sin – and use a warmer setting for styling. Point the dryer down the hairshaft and move the nozzle along with your brush. Finish each section with a blast of cool air, to close the cuticles.

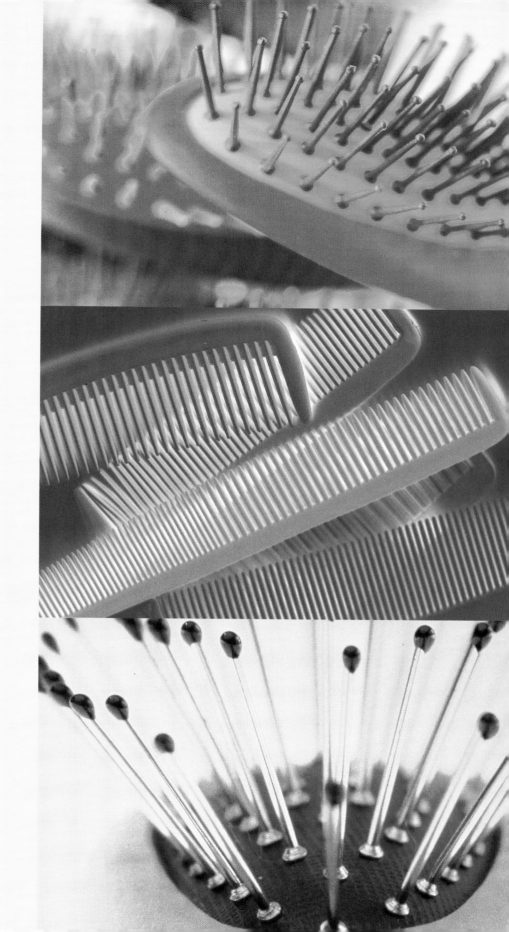

boost your brain power

Stress can dull even the sharpest mind. Unaddressed, stress can physically damage your brain and sap your energy. Most of the damage is wreaked by cortisol, one of the hormones secreted in response to stress. In moderate amounts it is not harmful, but when it is produced in excess, day after day, it is toxic enough to kill brain cells by the billion! The key is to set regular time aside for relaxation, which is the best way to boost mental energy. Try each of these exercises at least once during the weekend.

Write yourself a new life script

Boost your vitality with some positive 'self'-talk. The unconscious mind will always follow the stronger of two thoughts. If you think 'I can't cope' or 'I'm too tired to cope', that is the reality you will create. Write down some positive thoughts, such as 'I *can* cope', 'I am full of energy' and 'I can direct my life the way I want it to be'. Then repeat your positive thoughts to yourself regularly.

Breathe and regenerate

Breathing exercises are a good way to revitalize the mind. Try the Breath of Fire, a yoga exercise that increases inner calm and stimulates nerves in the abdominal cavity, causing the release of energy-boosting noradrenaline.
Inhale and exhale rapidly through your nostrils, without pausing between breaths. Concentrate on keeping your chest relaxed, and feel your diaphragm moving up and down with the breaths. You may feel light-headed but don't worry. The Breath of Fire produces relaxing alpha waves in the brain and also increases the level of oxygen in your blood, increasing mental alertness.

Watch a funny movie

This weekend set aside time to watch a video of your favourite comedy film – anything that you can rely on to give you a really good laugh! According to some experts, laughter is like 'stationary jogging', or 'internal aerobics'; a good hearty belly laugh has similar invigorating effects to going to the gym. It lowers your blood pressure, relaxes muscle tension, boosts your immune system and releases feel-good endorphins. It's one of the most enjoyable ways to pep you up and increase your energy levels!

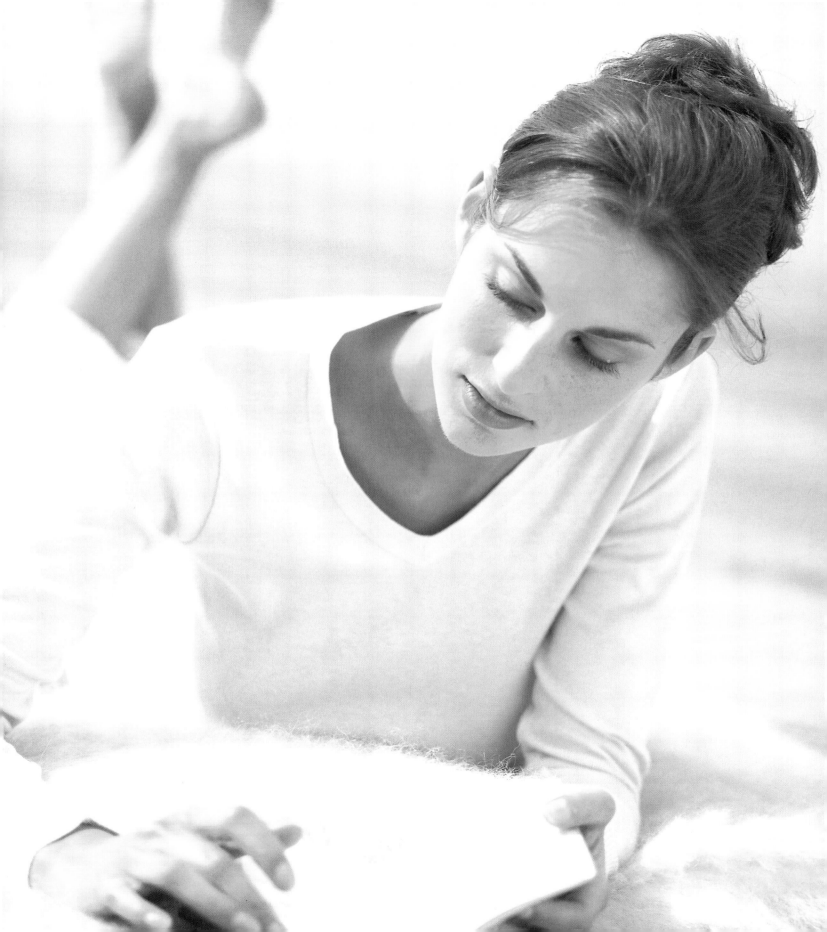

brain teasers

If you're lacking in mental energy, you may simply need to exercise your neglected grey matter with some brain exercise. Read a new novel, or try a crossword – remember the more you use your brain, the more adept it will be.

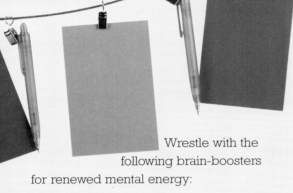

Wrestle with the following brain-boosters for renewed mental energy:

● Think of 20 words beginning with 'B' within 30 seconds.

● Within 30 seconds find an opposite for each of the following words: massive, weak, next, failure, fat, happy, lively, critical, open, clumsy.

● Within 60 seconds, find a word that means the same as each of the following words: chatty, finish, book, clean, ship, wealth, argue, obscurity, habit.

● Read the following eight words out loud twice: sun, vitamin, table, orange, pencil, horse, fruit, joy. Now close your eyes, say the alphabet backwards and then try to remember the words in the correct order.

energy moves

Energy flows best when you are relaxed and your mind, body and spirit are at one. The ancient discipline of t'ai chi is designed to encourage the flow of chi (or energy) in the body. Try this move from the Yang form of t'ai chi called 'wave hands like clouds'.

Carry out each exercise slowly in order to perfect your technique. Then, when you have mastered the technique, increase the speed and concentrate on your breathing. Use the minimum of muscular effort as tension inhibits chi flow. Practise the move regularly – either in the morning or at the end of the day.

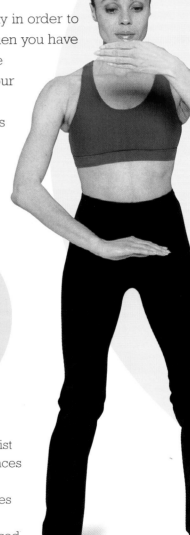

1 Stand with your feet shoulder-width apart, and your weight centred.

Body: keep your body relaxed and upright
Right arm: bring your forearm in front of you at hip height
Right wrist: flex your wrist
Right hand: your palm faces down
Left hand: your palm faces you
Left arm: your arm is raised
Knees: keep your knees slightly bent

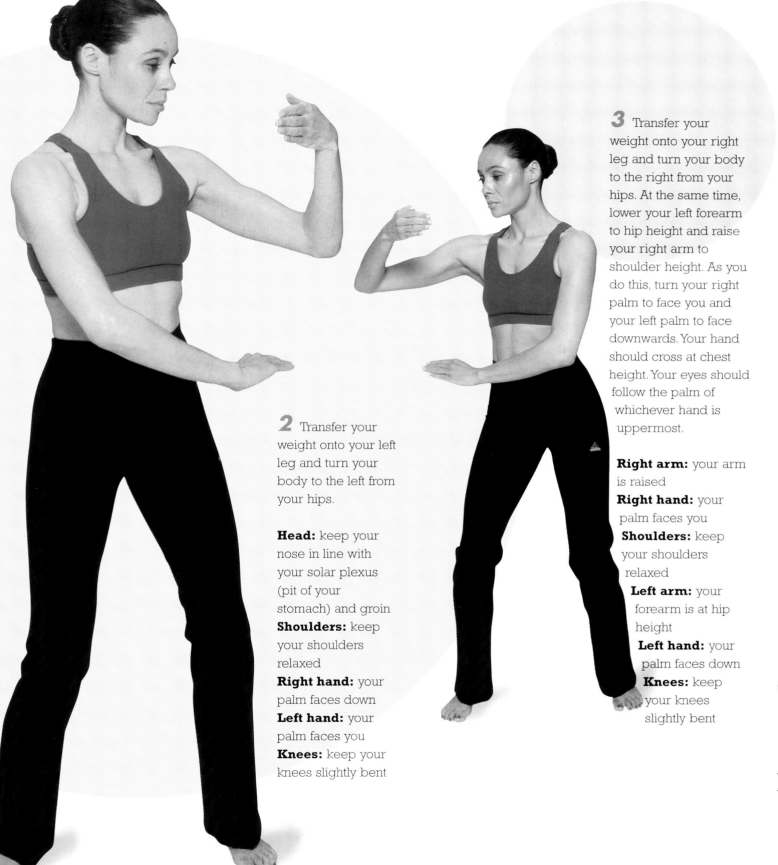

2 Transfer your weight onto your left leg and turn your body to the left from your hips.

Head: keep your nose in line with your solar plexus (pit of your stomach) and groin
Shoulders: keep your shoulders relaxed
Right hand: your palm faces down
Left hand: your palm faces you
Knees: keep your knees slightly bent

3 Transfer your weight onto your right leg and turn your body to the right from your hips. At the same time, lower your left forearm to hip height and raise your right arm to shoulder height. As you do this, turn your right palm to face you and your left palm to face downwards. Your hand should cross at chest height. Your eyes should follow the palm of whichever hand is uppermost.

Right arm: your arm is raised
Right hand: your palm faces you
Shoulders: keep your shoulders relaxed
Left arm: your forearm is at hip height
Left hand: your palm faces down
Knees: keep your knees slightly bent

CHAPTER 4

relaxing
Spa

rest and revive your body and mind

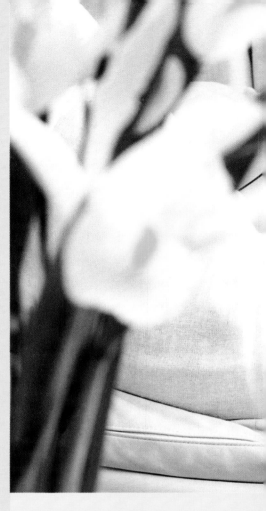

There's more to relaxing than being horizontal – although that's a good place to start! Sleep, good nutrition, simple relaxation exercises and meditations are all vital tools for restoring your equilibrium. And a little pampering can certainly imbue you with confidence and energy. So if you've been guilty of self-neglect of late, and wish to focus on resting your weary mind and body, read on.

EAT YOUR WAY TO RELAXATION

Certain foods can help you to relax. Carbohydrate-rich foods are the best fuel to soothe and nourish the body. For a weekend of complete relaxation eat small, regular meals, and foods that are easy to prepare and satisfying to eat. Eating carbohydrates regularly, while limiting stimulants such as caffeine, can help the calming process along.

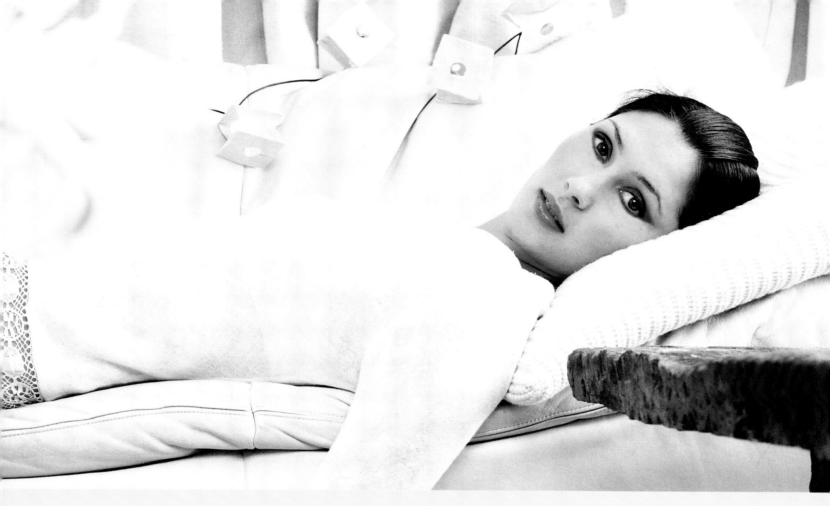

Choose Relaxing Foods

● Carbohydrate-rich meals can help you to feel calmer and improve your mood by increasing levels of serotonin, a mood-controlling 'messenger' in the brain.

● Vitamin B6 is needed to make serotonin, and is found in red meat, fish, chicken, potatoes, nuts, bananas, wholegrain breads and cereals, and vegetables.

● Magnesium, folic acid and vitamin B12 are required to manufacture dopamine, another mood managing chemical messenger. B12 is found in all animal products, plus fortified foods such as breakfast cereals and yeast extracts (which supply folic acid too). Magnesium and folic acid are found in green vegetables, nuts, pulses, potatoes and wholegrain bread.

● If you are a regular caffeine drinker, cut down rather than cut it out, as sudden withdrawal from this stimulant can leave you feeling headachey, irritable and not relaxed! Alternate caffeine with your favourite herbal or fruit tea.

MEAL IDEAS FOR MAXIMUM RELAXATION

Saturday

Breakfast: Fortified breakfast cereal with milk; banana

Snack: Wholemeal fruit scone

Lunch: Ham/chicken/fish granary bap with green salad

Snack: Dried fruit and nuts

Dinner: Roast chicken with sweet and standard potatoes, broccoli, green beans

Snack: Rice pudding with cinnamon and raisins or light chocolate mousse

Sunday

Breakfast: Cinnamon and raisin bagel with low fat soft cheese; orange juice

Snack: Banana

Lunch: Jacket potato with your favourite filling; mixed green leaves

Snack: Small pitta bread with houmus

Dinner: Stir-fried beef with green and red peppers and black bean sauce; boiled rice

Snack: Pineapple brûlée (Half fill a ramekin with fresh or canned pineapple, cover it with fromage frais and a drop of vanilla essence; sprinkle with 1 tablespoon of brown sugar and grill until sugar bubbles. Chill the brûlée before eating.)

relaxing yoga moves

the best prescription for a worn-out body is gentle mind and body exercise. Yoga is an ideal workout. It's gentle, easy to follow, and, even if it is the only form of exercise you have time to do, it still gives you a good workout.

Yoga is an excellent way to tone your body while calming your mind. It may not look like it's doing a lot, because it is an internal process. If you have never tried yoga before don't be disheartened, because it can be hard at first, however fit you are. Don't force your body into the poses. Instead use your breathing to help unlock any stiffness and move your body fluidly into the positions.

Breathing effectively is the key to yoga's effectiveness. Yoga teaches you to breathe through your nose and from your diaphragm, allowing your lungs to expand to their full capacity and forcing extra oxygen into your bloodstream. The breathing acts as a natural tranquilizer on your nervous system. Just five minutes can deeply relax you.

The quality of breathing, say yoga experts, is more important even than the quantity of your movement. If it's smooth, calm, soft and consistent you will fill your mind with clear alertness. People sometimes hold their breath when challenged in a certain yoga movement but it's important to try to avoid this. Let your breath flow freely. Breathe out and you'll find you can go deeper into the positions.

power yoga

Yoga can also make you strong and toned, and improve your cardiovascular and muscular stamina. The increasingly popular astanga (also known as power or dynamic yoga) is based on the same deep breathing techniques of other forms of yoga, but the movements are fast paced, almost athletic, and performed in a non-stop sequence. Devotees claim it is more effective than a weights routine and as good for the heart as running. It could really transform your shape.

This weekend begin with a simple, gentle 10-minute yoga workout. After the weekend, try to do it every day. You should feel your stress levels dissolve, your body relax and your energy levels soar. And you will be ready to progress to power yoga before you know it.

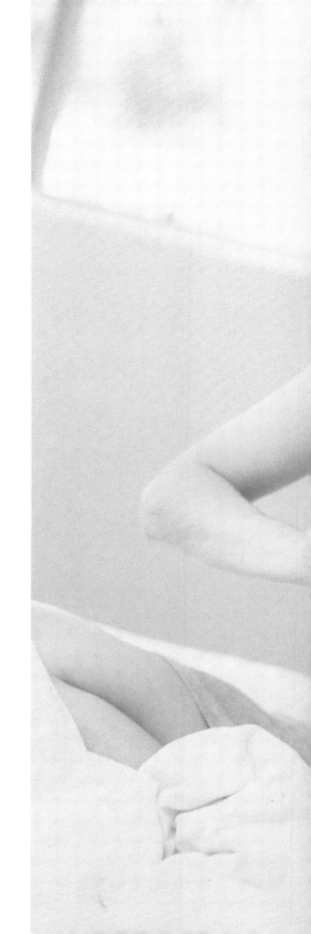

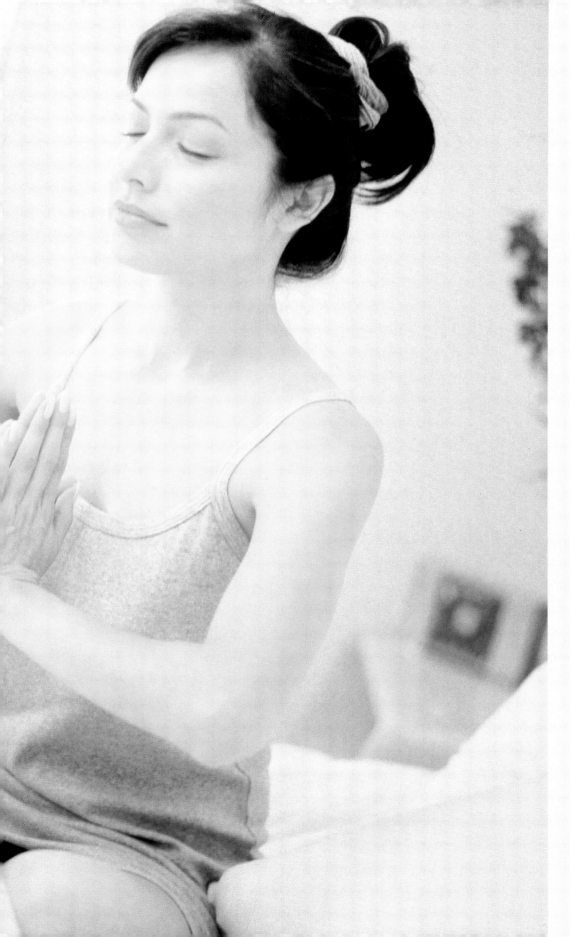

Before you start:

● Wear comfortable, loose clothing and find a place where you won't be disturbed. You may like to put on some relaxing music.

● Begin each pose by standing with your feet together and your arms by your sides.

● Do all the moves in the order given and bear in mind that all your movements should be smooth and fluid. Try to remember at all times to keep your hips square, your legs straight, and your spine 'long'.

● Don't forget that your breathing is vital. Focus on your breath all the time and try to bring real calm and stillness to your mind.

Exercises begin on following page

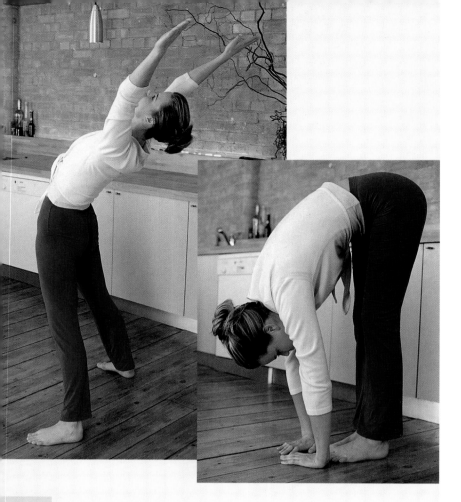

The ultimate stretch
For: Balance, focus, stamina and flexibility

1 Lift your right leg up behind you, holding your foot with your right hand.

2 Point your right toes and extend your left arm up, close to your ear. To help you balance, focus on a point in front of you. Hold for three to five seconds, breathing in and out until you feel you have achieved perfect balance.

3 Slowly lift your right leg as far behind you as possible. Bring your bodyweight forward, taking your left arm out in front. Keep your shoulders down. Hold for as long as is comfortable, breathing normally. Repeat the whole move on the other leg.

The energizer
For: A deep stretch and better breath control

1 Stand with your feet slightly wider than shoulder-width apart. Hold your arms down in front of you, with your palms touching your thighs. Inhale deeply and bend backwards, extending your arms above your head as you do so. Push your hips as far forward as you can, and bend as far back as is comfortable for you. Hold this position for a slow count of three, without exhaling.

2 Exhale and, stretching forwards from your tailbone, bring your spine down and your body forwards so your palms touch the floor. If you can't reach the floor, bend your knees. Hold and breathe deeply for five to seven seconds.

3 Inhale and slowly uncurl your spine, returning to a standing posture. Repeat from the beginning, five times.

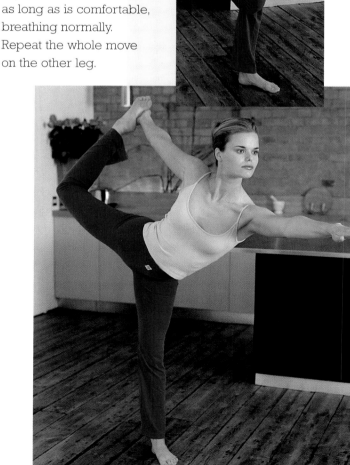

The stress reliever

For: Release of tension in the spine, neck and shoulders

1 Kneel with your knees hip-width apart. Keeping your spine straight, lightly hold your forearms behind your back. Inhale deeply. Exhale and push your hips as far forwards as you can.

2 Grasp your heels. If you can't reach, keep holding your arms. Relax your head and neck back to create an arch, and hold for five to seven seconds, breathing deeply.

3 Slowly sit down on your heels. Move your body forwards until you're resting your forehead on the floor. Hold for five to seven seconds. Repeat once.

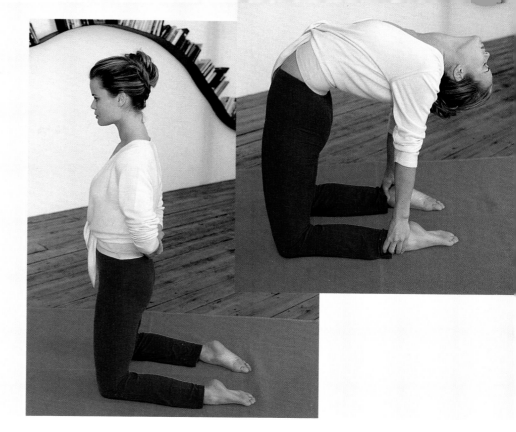

The deep relaxer

For: Relaxation of every muscle in the body

1 Sit with your knees together and your bottom between your feet. With your hands resting on your feet, start to lower your body backwards onto your elbows.

2 When you feel comfortable, lie back all the way and take your hands over your head, resting them on your forearms. If you feel any discomfort, put a pillow under the small of your back. Take very deep breaths and focus on your breathing for as long as you can – aim for five minutes.

3 Slowly return to the starting position by pushing your chest forward, going back onto your elbows, then using your stomach muscles to push yourself up. Do this move once only.

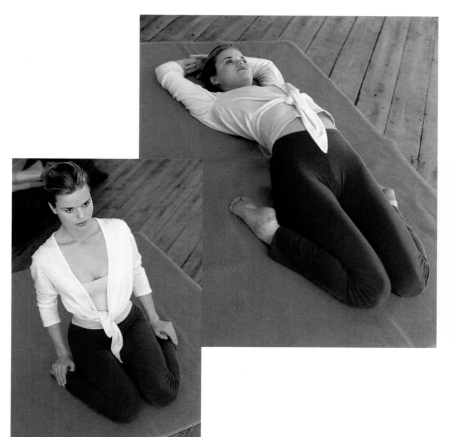

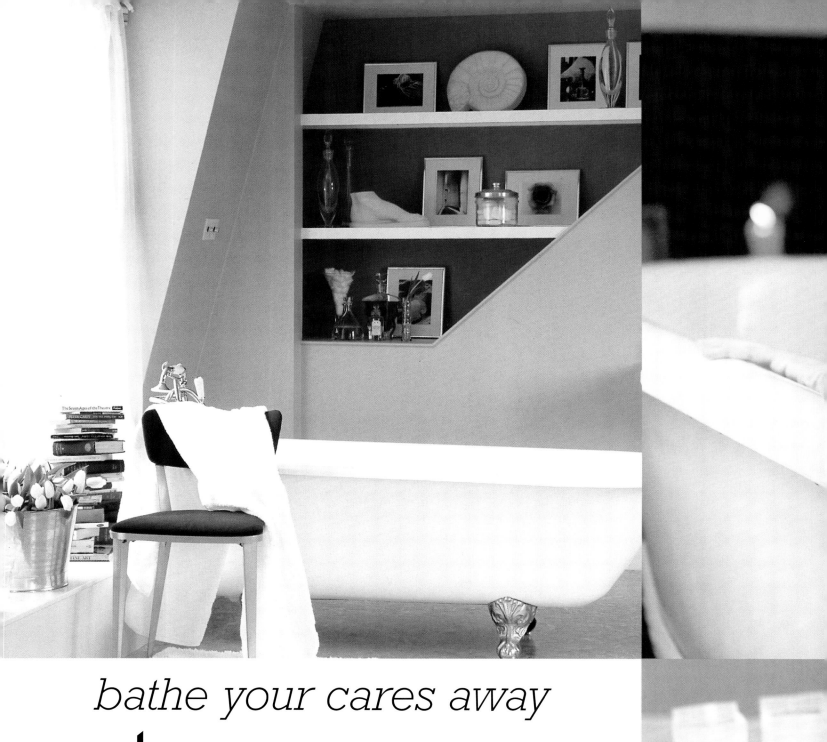

bathe your cares away

the bath is the ideal place to dissolve your troubles because the ritual of bathing involves so much more than getting clean. Bathtime is thinking time, relaxing time, daydreaming time. Your bath can be a place of rejuvenation, relaxation and beautification. You just need the right props and a little time to spare. If you wish, you can preface your bath with a thorough facial (see page 31), or just slap on a face mask and slip into the tub.

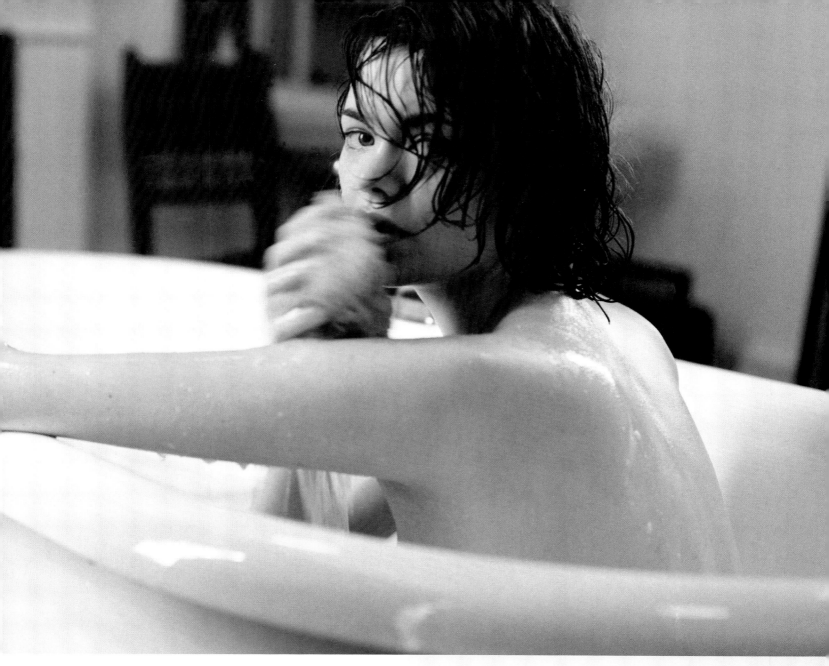

create the ambience

Think mellow. Declutter the bathroom, have a battery-operated CD player at hand for soothing sounds, light some scented candles, The trick is to really wallow in your bath. Add bubbles, oils, rose petals... whatever you wish.

Concoct your own relaxing blend of essential oils to use in a nightlight diffuser. Pre-mix 15 to 20 drops of oil in a 100 to 125 ml bottle of water and fill the reservoir with a little of the blend (shake the bottle a little each time). Three or four drops is usually enough for an average-sized room.

Oils for the bath Dilute five or six drops of essential oil in milk or vodka (both act as a dispersant), and sprinkle the mixture over the bath's surface. Make sure the water is not too hot or the oils will evaporate. Limit your bathing time to 20 minutes, after which your skin will start to shrivel!

Soak, relax and breathe in the aroma. If you suffer from dry skin, dilute the pure essential oil in 10 ml of a carrier oil, such as almond or grapeseed oil, which has moisturizing properties.

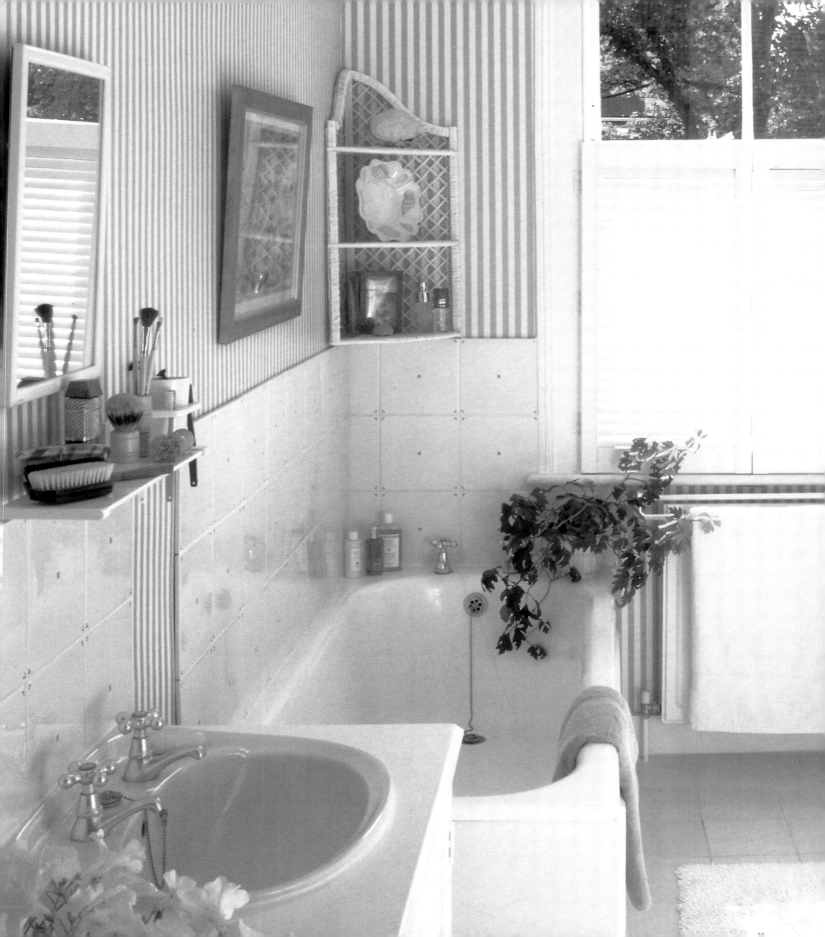

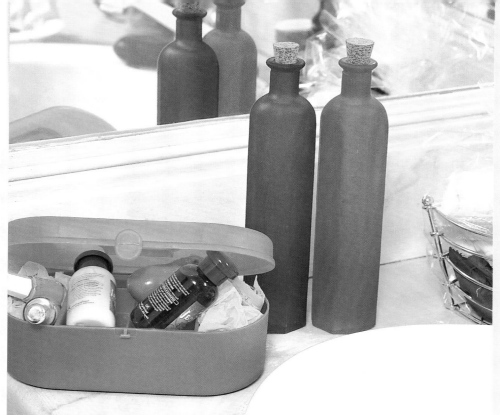

bathtime breathing

As you soak, try to relax your body. Take slow deep breaths through your nostrils and focus on your diaphragm as it moves up and down. As a guide, you should aim to take four seconds to breathe in and four seconds to breathe out. Then try to let go of each muscle area, until you've covered your entire body. Mentally scan your body for tense points, exaggerate their tension to an unbearable degree, then let go.

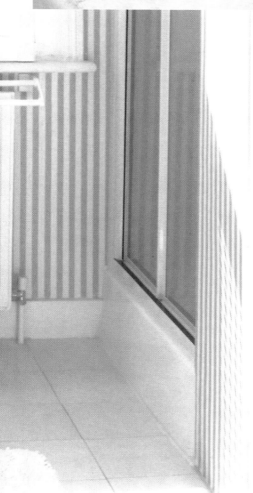

aromatherapy relaxation oils

Certain aromatherapy oils have properties to help the relaxation process. The smells influence your mental attitude because the olfactory area of the brain is closely connected to the areas dealing with emotion, intuition and creativity. Mix the oils in equal quantities.

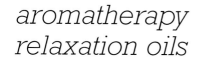

for relaxation:
● cypress, juniper and pine
● bergamot, grapefruit, lemon, lime, mandarin and orange
● clary sage, geranium, lavender, neroli and petitgrain

for sleep:
● camomile, clary sage and lavender
● frankincense, patchouli, vetiver or sandalwood
● neroli, rose otto and ylang ylang

for a relaxing wallow:
● **bergamot** (antiseptic, relaxing, uplifting)
● **clary sage** (antiseptic, soothing, relaxing, balancing)
● **cypress** (antiseptic, balancing, relaxing, a tonic)
● **frankincense** (antiseptic, balancing, relaxing, a tonic)
● **lavender** (comforting, restorative)
● **mandarin** (relaxing)
● **myrrh** (antiseptic, relaxing, soothing)
● **Roman chamomile** (relaxing, antiseptic)
● **sweet marjoram** (antiseptic, relaxing, warming, a tonic)
● **ylang ylang** (soothing, balancing, comforting)

(Never use essential oils on children, or if you are pregnant, without first consulting a qualified aromatherapist.)

acupressure

acupressure is a simple hands-on therapy that boosts your body, and relaxes and revitalizes your mind. It is based on the premise that everyone has a vital force of energy that flows along established channels, or meridians, which are connected to different organs and body systems. If this flow of energy is interrupted, by stress for example, it creates an imbalance within your body that manifests itself on the outside. By stimulating certain points that lie beneath the surface of the skin (the acupressure points) you can restore your body's natural harmony.

BEFORE YOU START

Acupressure is very safe. Even if you have difficulty finding an acupressure point and end up applying pressure in the wrong place, you will not do yourself any harm. However, take the following precautions:
● avoid acupressure treatment on open wounds, varicose veins, bruised, broken or inflamed skin
● if you are pregnant avoid the following points: large intestine 4, urinary bladder 60
● avoid treatment if you are under the influence of drink or recreational drugs

How to apply the pressure:

● When you have found the right point, you may feel a mild pain sensation. Sometimes you may find it more effective to position your thumb or fingertip at an angle to the point.
● Apply deep pressure on each acupoint for about one second, then release it. Continue with this 'pumping' action for one minute.
● Don't apply prolonged pressure on the various acupoints because the nerves that carry out the therapeutic impulses may become overaccustomed to the stimulus.

movements to try during your relaxation weekend

For emotional balance:

Name of acupoint? extra point 6
Where is it? Two finger-widths to the left and the right of GV20 (see page 70), which is in the middle of the top of your head. Apply pressure with the index and middle finger of each hand.
What does it do? Balances the mind and emotions. Relieves anxiety and insomnia. Use whenever the need arises.

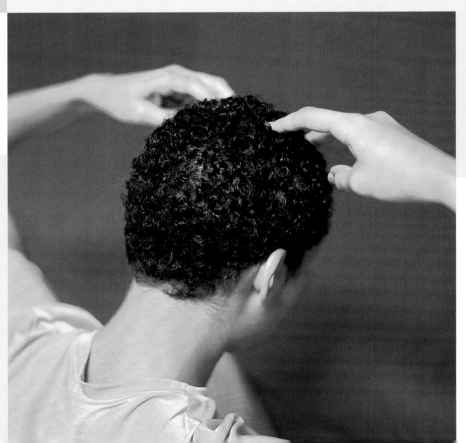

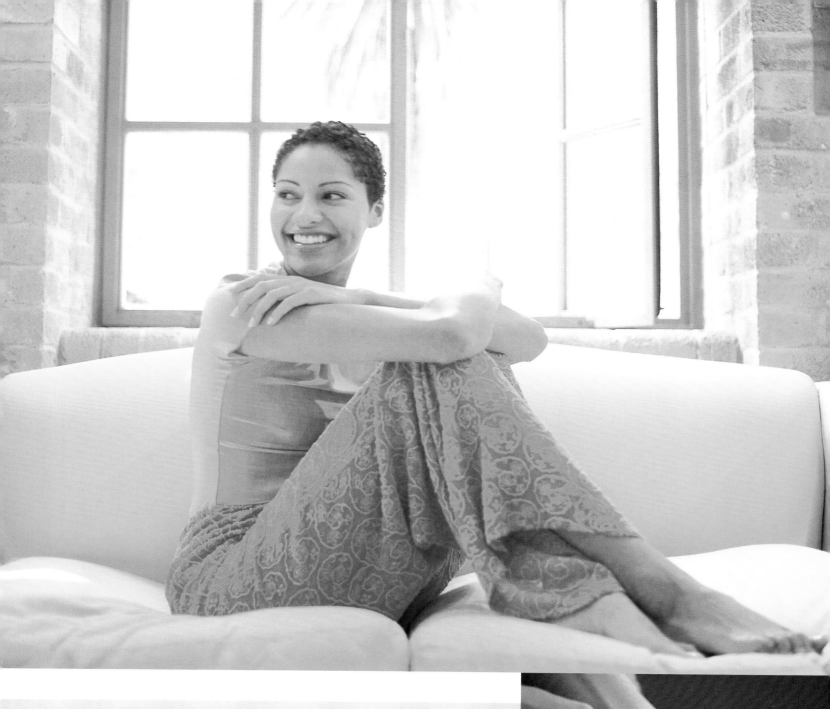

For overall wellbeing:

Name of acupoint? urinary
bladder 60 (UB60)

Where is it? On the outer side of
the foot, in the hollow between the
ankle bone and your Achilles
tendon. Apply pressure with your
index finger (do not stimulate the
point when pregnant).

What does it do? Boosts your
immune system and the functioning
of your urinary system. Increases
mobility and relieves pain and
swelling in legs, ankles and feet.

Continued next page

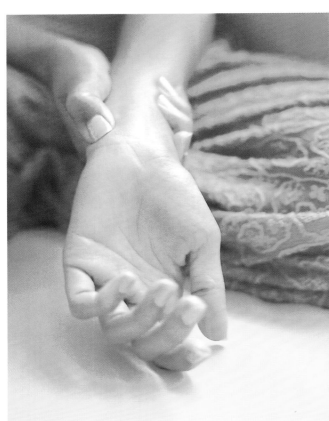

For a better night's sleep:

Name of acupoint? heart 7 (Ht7)

Where is it? With your palm facing up, draw an imaginary line from between your ring and little fingers to your wrist. Ht 7 lies at the junction of this line and the wrist crease. Support your wrist in the opposite hand and apply pressure with thumb.

What does it do? Relieves anxiety and sleeplessness. Calms the nervous system. Helpful if you are trying to give up smoking.

For clear thinking:

Name of acupoint? governing vessel 20 (GV20)

Where is it? It's situated in the middle of the top of your head, halfway between your ears. Apply pressure using your index finger.

What does it do? This is the most powerful sedative point in the body. It balances the emotions and sharpens your mental faculties as well as improving your memory and concentration. It's also very effective at regulating blood pressure and raising your general energy levels.

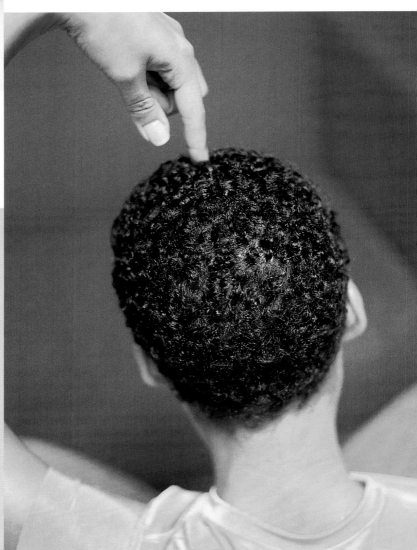

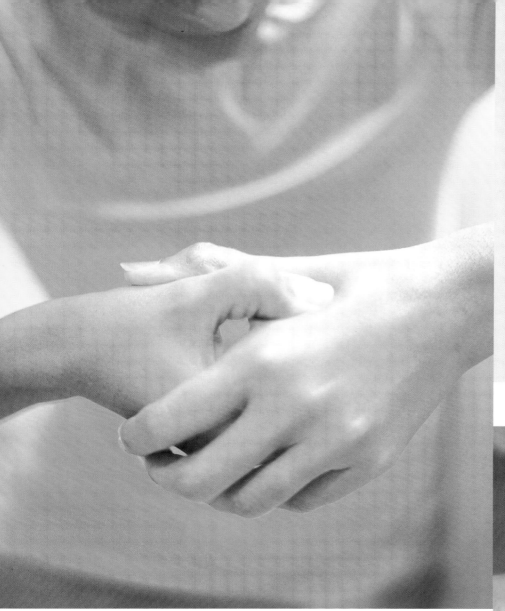

For headache-free calm:

Name of acupoint? large intestine 4 (LI4)

Where is it? At the peak of the mound of muscle created when you press your thumb and index fingers together. Apply pressure with your other thumb. (Do not stimulate this point when pregnant.)

What does it do? Sometimes referred to as the 'aspirin' point, this is effective at treating problems affecting the front of the head, the face (including the sense organs) and the neck. Calms the mind, relaxes the upper body and relieves tension in the neck, shoulders, arms and hands. Enhances mental function. Regulates function of lower intestine. Promotes elimination of toxins.

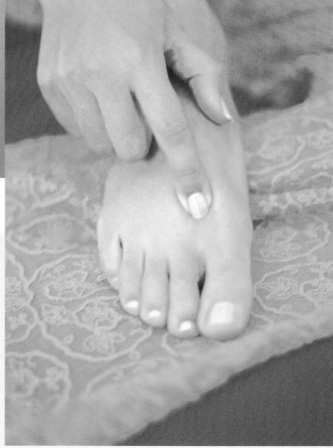

For a more positive outlook:

Name of acupoint? liver 3 (Liv 3)

Where is it? On the upper part of your foot, about two thumb widths below the web between the big toe and the second toe. Use your index finger to apply pressure in the hollow between the bones.

What does it do? Improves liver function, boosts the immune system and reduces irritability (sometimes called liverishness). Combats depression. Relieves the effects of stress and toxins on the body and regulates blood pressure. Boosts circulation in the legs, relieves cramp and helps prevent varicose veins.

delicious, beautifying sleep

Do you want to look and feel relaxed? Really relaxed? There is nothing more nourishing and revitalizing than sleep. The problem is that we sometimes lose the knack of getting to sleep. This weekend you are going to sleep yourself back to vitality, by brushing up on your slumber 'hygiene', which means ensuring your bedtime habits and your bedroom itself encourage sleep.

Your guide to restful sleep

● Create the perfect bedroom
Your bedroom should be comfortable (neither too hot nor too cold), dark, quiet and free from reminders of work. Try not to watch television or eat in bed. Reserve your bed for sleep.

● Reset your sleep/wake cycle
Get up at the same time every day until your body's circadian (natural) rhythm has been restored. Even if you have been sleeping badly, try to sacrifice a lie-in this weekend. Don't expect to feel rested if you force yourself to sleep until lunchtime on Saturday or Sunday because daylight tells your brain that it is time to wake up. This is because the sleep/wake cycle is governed by the hormone melatonin, which is sensitive to light and dark.

● Don't sleep too long
You can actually sleep too much; sleep consists of 90-minute cycles of both light and deep sleep. After a normal night's sleep your body wakes up naturally, usually coinciding with the end of a 90-minute sleep cycle. If you extend your sleeping hours, you risk waking up during the next cycle's deep phase from which it is often harder to surface. This can make you feel groggy and disorientated.

● Avoid rich food at night
Don't go to bed after a heavy meal (wait about two hours) or on an empty stomach (have a light snack such as cereal or a milky drink).

● Adopt a new sleep position
The Chinese believe you should sleep on your right side, almost in a foetal position with your legs slightly bent and your right arm resting in front of the pillow to allow your blood to circulate freely.

● Use lavender oil
Lavender is a well-established traditional remedy for insomnia, and lavender essential oil has now been scientifically proven to have a sedative effect on the brain. Put a few drops on your pillow.

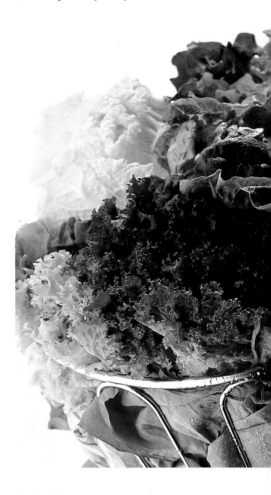

● Eat lettuce
The natural sleep-inducing properties of lettuce are believed to be the reason why pet tortoises, whose diet is largely made up of lettuce, sleep so much! Lettuce contains tryptophan, which triggers the production of the calming brain chemical serotonin.

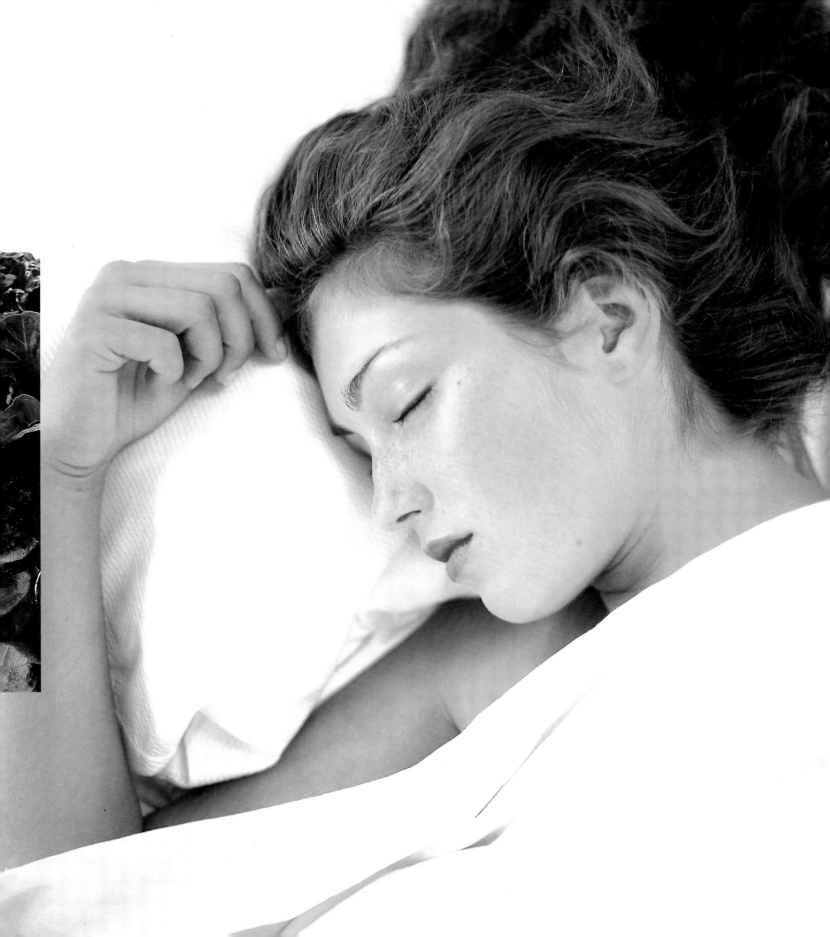

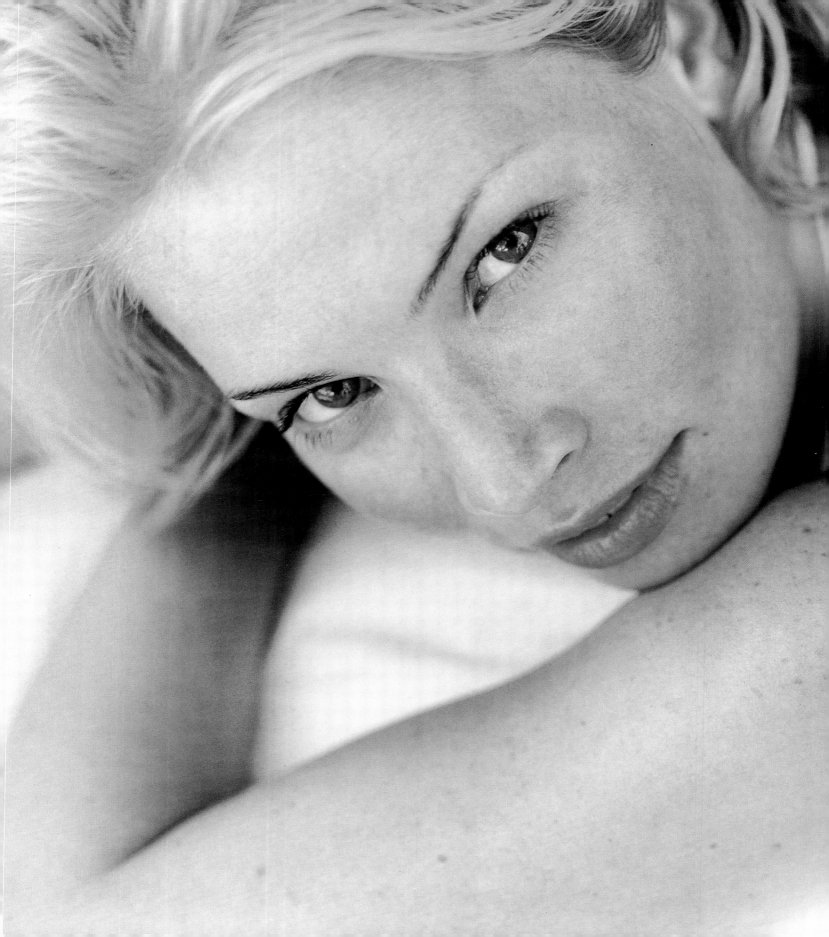

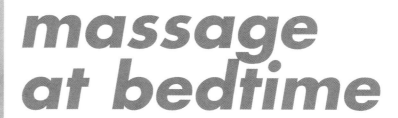

massage at bedtime

During sleep, cell-renewal doubles and general rejuvenation kicks in. A good night's sleep will also relax your facial muscles so that by the time you wake up in the morning, lines, bags and shadows can almost be soothed away. Try the following intensive relaxing evening treatment during your Relaxing Spa weekend to promote a good night's sleep, bolster your moisture levels and relieve tired, stressed skin.

1 Take a warm bath doused with relaxing oils to unwind. (Your whole body needs to be relaxed for your skin to benefit.)

2 Practise 'abdominal breathing' (long, slow deep breaths that fill your lungs right down to the bottom) to relax your mind.

3 Give yourself a five-minute pressure-point massage with a gentle facial oil. Move the tips of your ring fingers in small, circular movements over your third eye (the space between your eyes above the bridge of your nose), your temples, the corners of your nose either side of your nostrils, the dimple of your chin, the corners of your mouth and back up to your temples. Repeat three times, massaging slightly more deeply each time.

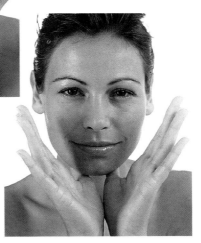

CHAPTER 5

pampering
Spa

glamour! decadence! luxury!

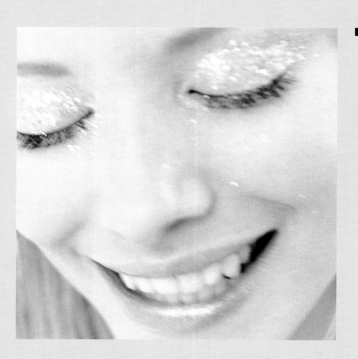

these are the ingredients of the Pampering Spa, designed for when you crave – or feel you deserve – some shameless, unadulterated pleasure. This weekend is about sheer hedonism. It will be a feast for your senses. If you want to work out and brush up, then incorporate a beauty treatment or an exercise programme into your weekend, as your energy or inclination take you. Alternatively, eat, drink and lounge around to your heart's desire – and rouse yourself only for a spell of serious glamourizing!

An epicurean weekend

It's your party, so feel free to help yourself to indulgent, pleasurable foods. But rather than eating to excess, take the time to touch, taste and savour your favourite treats. You can indulge, without overdosing on fats. Think fresh mangoes, seafood, pistachios, a glass of champagne, a nibble of the finest chocolate, the freshest pasta, sun-ripened tomatoes. Treat yourself this weekend, but focus on eating the foods you really enjoy; feel satisfied but don't overdo it!

Pampering foods:

● Before the weekend, make a list of what you really enjoy eating. Concentrate on taste, texture, aroma, satisfaction; quality not quantity.

● Choose a variety of foodstuffs to keep your diet balanced, such as seafood or meats, crusty continental breads, fresh, filled pasta, wild, nutty rice, goat's cheese, vine tomatoes, basil, olive oil, lychees, fresh figs, chocolate, champagne.

● Only eat when you feel truly hungry. Stop as soon as you feel satisfied. Try to maintain a 'food for satisfaction' philosophy after the weekend is over.

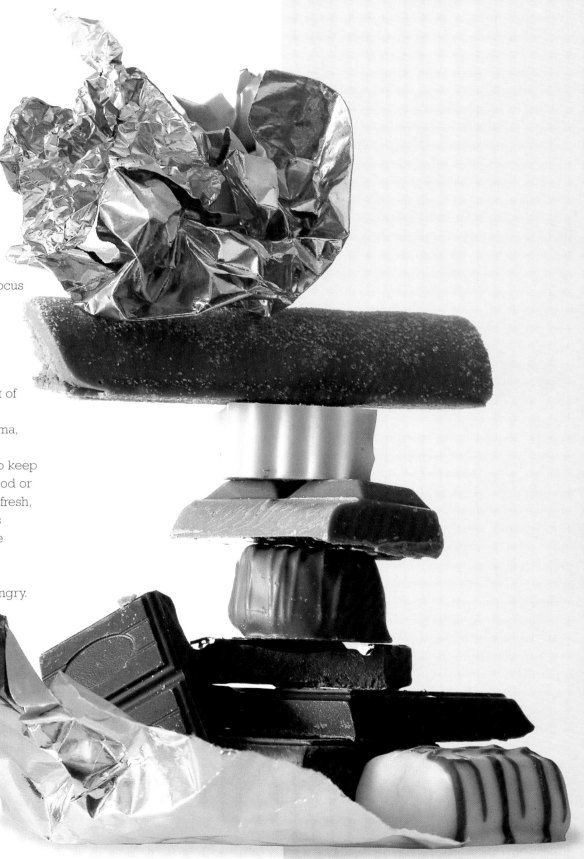

Sinful but saintly

You can electrify your tastebuds without increasing the size of your thighs. With some clever low-fat improvization, traditional high-fat, high-calorie foods can be transformed into healthy (or healthy-ish) indulgences.

Fruit brûlée

Makes two

This amounts to a mere 168 calories and 0.16 percent fat per serving, plus it's a good source of potassium and vitamins A and C. Also a good source of calcium and fibre.

50 g (2 oz) fresh, ripe strawberries
40 g (1½ oz) fresh raspberries
25 g (1 oz) caster sugar
1 small ripe but firm peach
1 small ripe mango
1 dessertspoon Kirsch (optional)
175 g (6 oz) natural virtually fat-free
  fromage frais

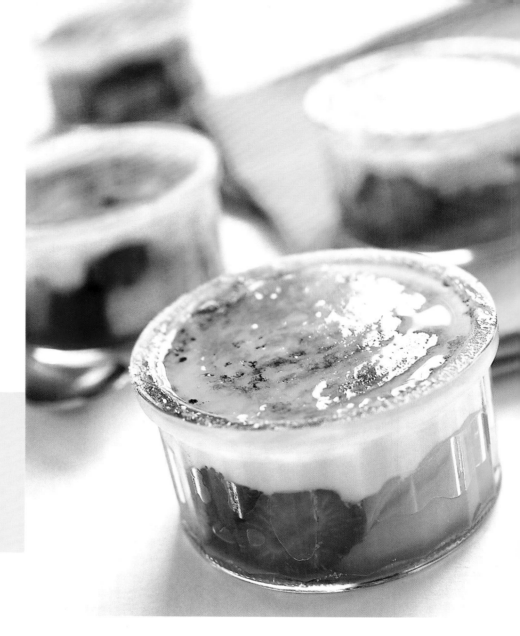

1 Wash, dry, hull and quarter the strawberries and put them in a bowl. Add the raspberries and sprinkle with 5 g (¼ oz) of the caster sugar. Mix gently together and set aside.

2 Halve and stone the peach and put it into a bowl. Cover with boiling water and leave to stand for 1 minute. Then drain, skin, and slice the peach halves and add them to the berry mixture.

3 Slice rounded slices off the mango's central stone and score the flesh deeply with a criss-cross

pattern. Hold each half with the flesh-side uppermost and press the skin with your thumbs to invert it and push out the flesh. Cut the rest of the mango from the skin and add to the other fruit. Sprinkle with the Kirsch, if using, and mix gently together.

4 Divide the prepared fruit between two 200 ml (8 fl oz) ramekin dishes or other small flameproof dishes. Spoon the fromage frais on top of the fruit and spread evenly over.

5 Sprinkle the remaining caster sugar over the top, then immediately caramelize the sugar with a cook's blowtorch. If you don't have a blowtorch, put the remaining sugar into a small saucepan with 1 dessertspoon cold water and stir over a moderate heat until the sugar is dissolved. Bring to the boil and continue boiling until the syrup turns a caramel colour. Quickly drizzle the caramel over the fromage frais. Chill the ramekins well, until ready to serve.

Strawberries in red wine

Two servings – eat one straightaway and keep one in the fridge for later.

114 calories and 0g fat per serving. Excellent source of vitamin C.

250 g (8 oz) fresh, ripe strawberries, washed, dried, hulled and at room temperature

finely zested rind of ¼ orange

20 g (¾ oz) fine, organic cane sugar

115 ml (4 fl oz) Cabernet Sauvignon red wine

a few strips of orange rind to decorate (optional)

1 Put the strawberries (whole if small, halved if large) into a bowl and add the zested orange rind.

Sprinkle with the sugar, add the red wine and stir gently together. Cover and leave to soak at room temperature for 20 to 30 minutes, stirring occasionally.

2 Spoon the mixture into wine glasses. Decorate with the strips of orange rind, if using, and eat. When you have finished the strawberries, just slurp the deliciously strawberry-flavoured wine straight from the glass.

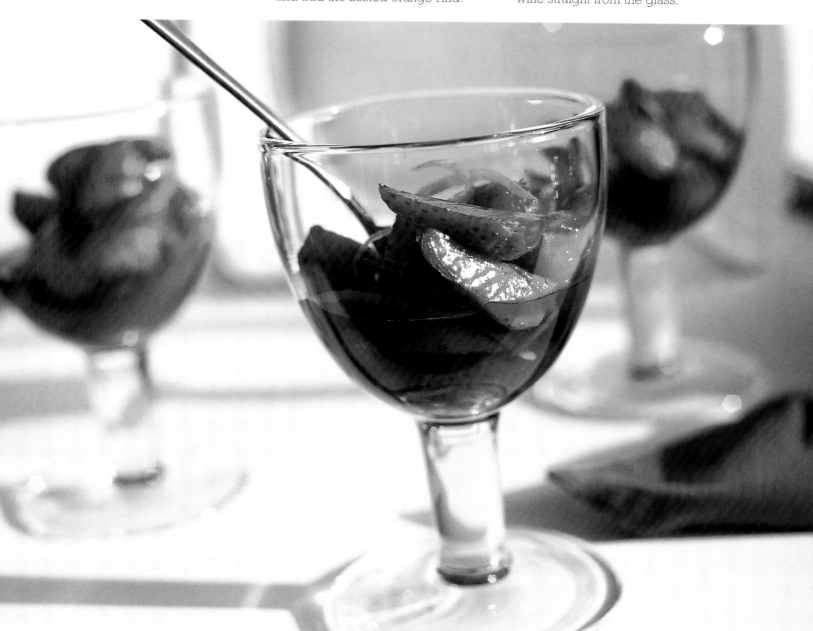

let go!

dancing queen

Few things impart a feel-good factor like dancing does. It's also a fantastic calorie burner. Did you know that moderate to vigorous dancing can burn nearly six calories a minute? Waltzing or rumba-ing your way around the room with a partner can burn as much as 420 calories an hour. Dancing in the privacy of your own home is also a great way to de-stress and 'express' yourself, whether you prefer twirling around Isadora Duncan-style, or high-kicking your way around the room. So this weekend, shut the door behind you, stick on a CD and let yourself go...

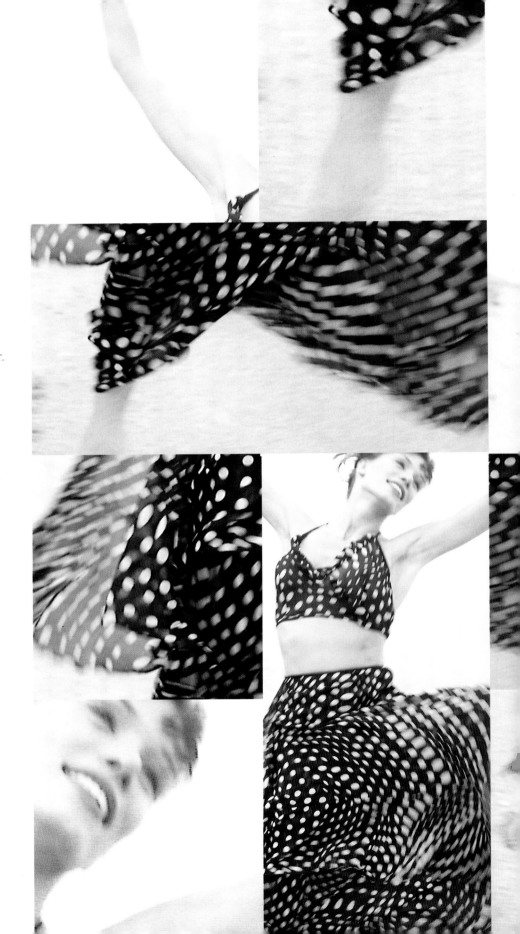

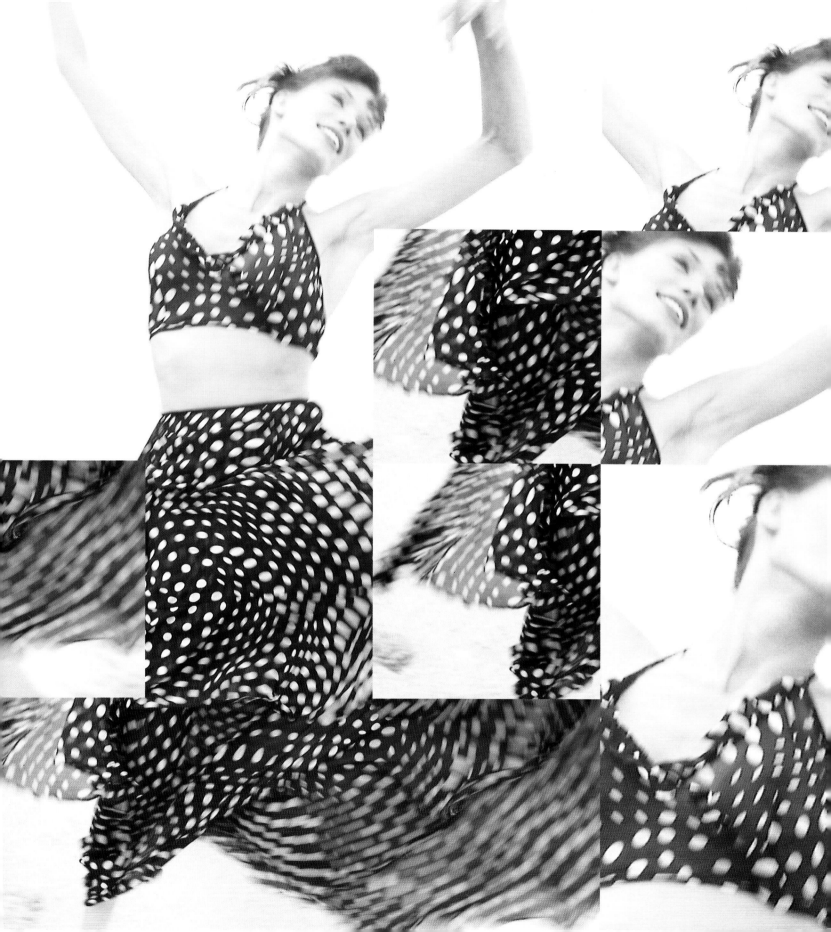

top to toe attention

there's nothing little girls like to do more than play at dressing up with the clothes, the hair, the make-up. Even for big girls it's still great fun, and there are added benefits – instant glamour, increased confidence, and head-turning gorgeousness. So pour yourself a glass of champagne, grab all your lotions and potions, dust off those grooming tools, and transform yourself from top to toe.

beautiful hair

Give yourself a salon-style treatment with a pre-wash scalp massage. The result? Head-turning hair.

1 Massage 1 teaspoon of a hair treatment oil (or culinary almond or olive oil) deeply into the scalp with the pads of your fingers, using a slow, kneading movement. Start at the front of your head and work backwards to the nape of your neck. Leave the oil to soak in for about 10 minutes, then shampoo your hair as normal with a mild shampoo.

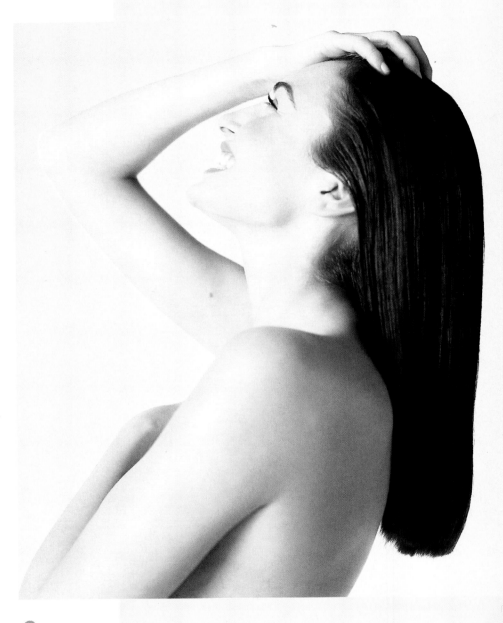

2 After rinsing, apply a conditioning treatment. Wrap a towel or clingfilm around your head to generate heat, which helps the conditioning treatment to penetrate more deeply into each hair shaft. Leave for about half an hour, then rinse well.

elegant, plucked eyebrows

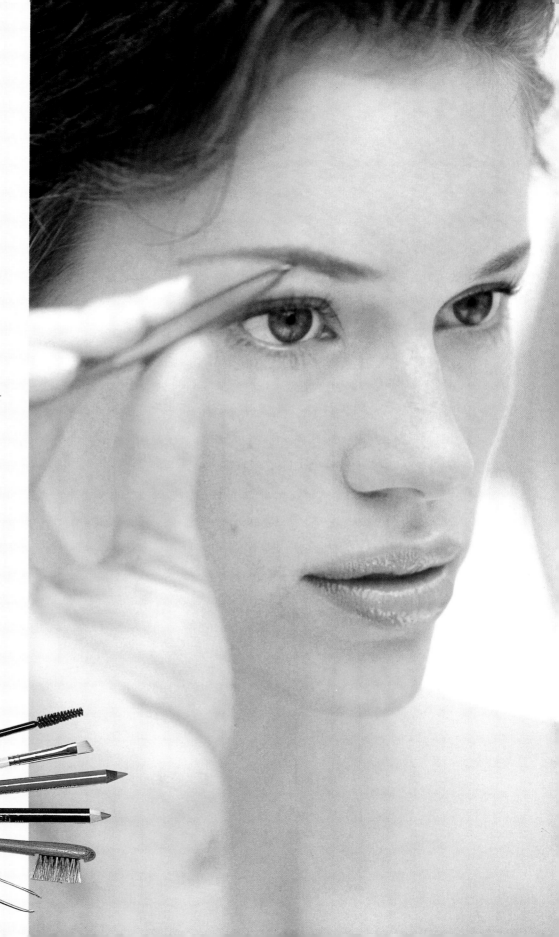

Plucking your eyebrows needn't hurt if you follow these pain-free steps.

1 Comb your brows in one direction, then the opposite way to dislodge any loose hairs.

2 Pull your skin taut with the thumb and index finger of one hand and hold the tweezers in the other hand with your fingers near the ends of the tweezers (but not touching the skin) for more plucking power.

3 Pluck the hairs one at a time, gripping them close to the root. Start with the hairs near the middle of your eyebrows and pluck only the stray hairs. Work in a line outwards towards your ears. Don't remove any hairs above the browline.

4 Have an ice cube to hand. After plucking each hair, place the ice over the area to tighten the pore and desensitize the skin.

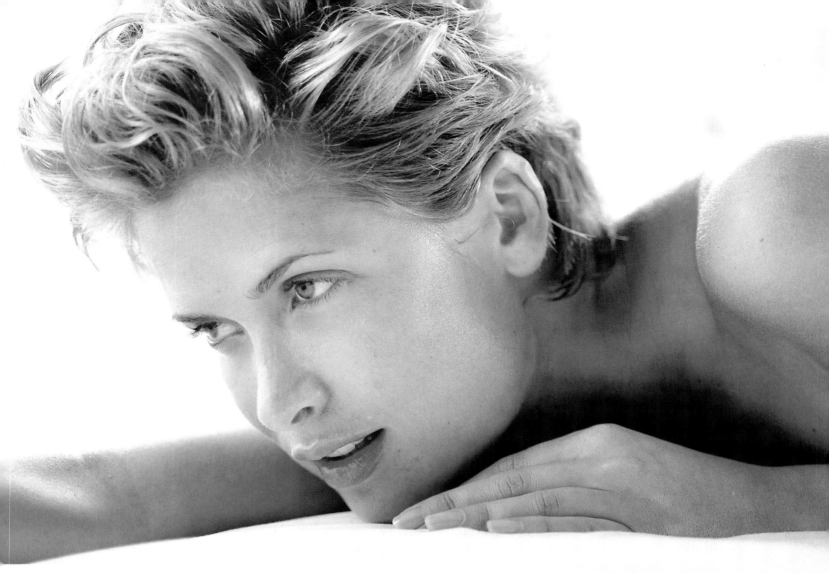

baby soft skin

Exfoliation is the key to getting rid of dry, flaky skin.

1 Take an exfoliating cream or scrub into the shower and work over your body in circular movements.

2 Alternatively, use Epsom salts (available from chemists' shops). Fill a cup with the salts and add enough water to make a paste. Gently massage the paste over your skin, then rinse it off. The salts will help to deep cleanse your skin (so you may find you sweat a lot afterwards).

3 Moisturize after exfoliating, or soak in a bath, or use aromatherapy oils to boost your skin and your mood.

A healthy holiday glow

Fake tan is the best and healthiest way to go bronze without risking sun damage. A light, sun-kissed looking tan can hide a multitude of nasties from flab to cellulite, while also making your limbs look longer.

1 For a seamless, streak-free tan, begin by exfoliating, then dry your skin. Moisturize only if your skin is extremely dry, then wait

magnificent nails

Neat, salon-style, manicured nails are the icing on the cake when it comes to grooming and glamour.

1 Remove old nail polish, then gently shape each nail with an emery board, using light strokes from the edges of the nail towards the centre.

2 Massage the cuticles with a little cuticle cream, or add a few drops of cuticle massage oil to a bowl of warm water. Soak the cuticles for five minutes. Then push them back using a cuticle stick. Wash your hands.

3 Apply a protective base coat of clear varnish, then a coat or two of colour, if required. Rest your hands for 20 minutes to avoid smudging. Finally, add a sealing top coat.

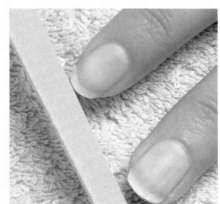

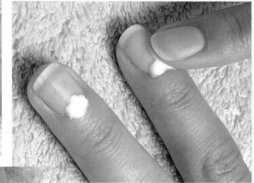

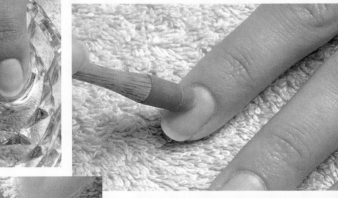

about 15 minutes for the cream to absorb – so that it doesn't interfere with the DHA (dihydroxacetone), which is the active ingredient in all tanning products.

2 Using a large make-up sponge, apply fake tan all over, blending and smoothing for an even coverage. Allow to dry for about 20 minutes.

3 To prevent your palms from being stained brown, rub them with fresh lemon juice.

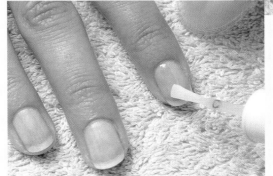

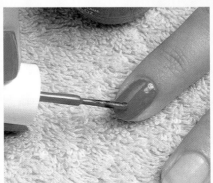

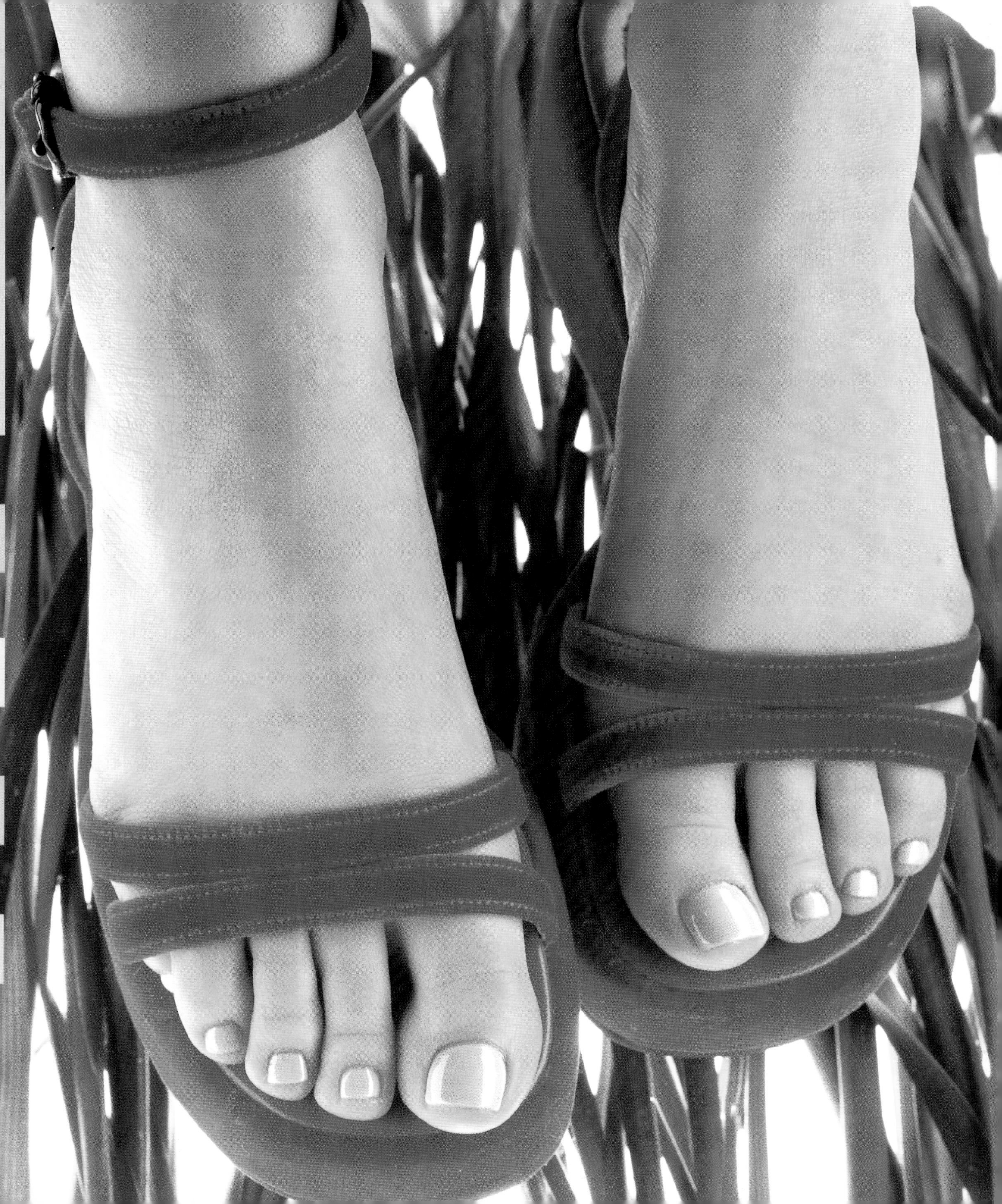

fabulous feet

Feet are rarely a woman's most treasured assets, and are often sorely neglected. A salon-style pedicure will transform and rejuvenate even the most unpleasant extremities, so get ready to pamper them.

1 Fill a foot bath with warm water to soften and hydrate your feet. While your feet are damp, gently buff away any hard skin using a pumice. (If you have very hard skin, dry your feet first, then use a buffer as it will be a lot more effective.)

2 Massage a foot scrub or exfoliating cream into your soles and rinse. Apply a thin layer of foot cream and wrap your feet in a towel or plastic bag for five to ten minutes, then rinse thoroughly. This will both soften and stimulate your feet.

3 Apply half a teaspoon of massage oil to your feet (try jojoba, sandalwood or ylang ylang oils diluted in carrier oil) and massage your feet using a twisting and kneading motion working from your toes to your knees. This is also a good time to push back your cuticles as they will be soft and pliable.

4 Give your nails a clean, healthy look by using a three-way nail buffer (available from chemists) to buff away any stains, and to add shine.

5 To remove bad stains, dissolve a couple of denture cleansing tablets in a glass of water, dip your nailbrush into it and gently scrub your nails. Make sure you give your hands a thorough, soapy wash afterwards.

6 Then finish off with a couple of layers of nail colour or clear lacquer.

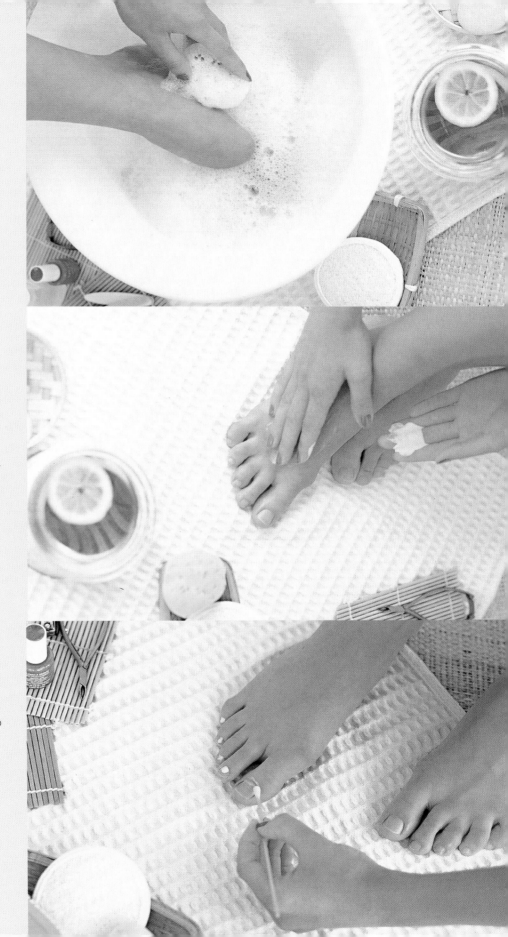

make-up tricks

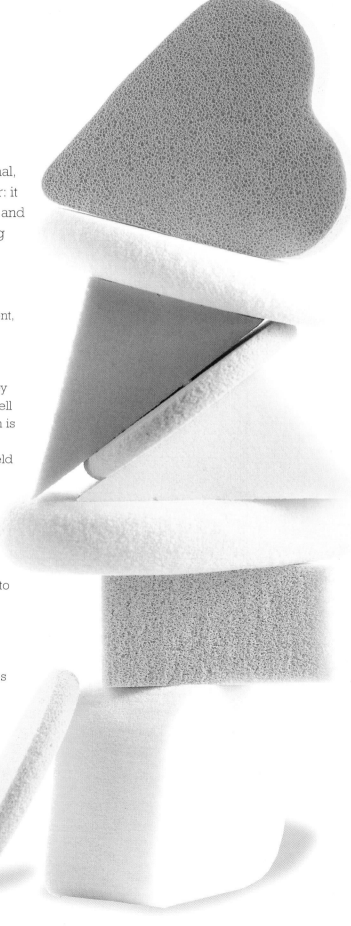

a vital component in any glamorous woman's arsenal, make-up is not only there to make you look better: it makes you feel powerful, boosts your confidence and protects your skin. Here are some great reasons for putting your best face forward.

● *It makes you feel good*
Make-up is like a self-protective armour. If you have the right front, you will have more confidence to present yourself as you want.

● *It protects your skin*
Most foundations not only give you a flawless make-up base, they also contain pollution-fighting and skin-firming ingredients, as well as sun protection factors and antioxidants. So wearing foundation is in itself anti-ageing because most contain pigments, such as titanium dioxide and iron oxide, which also act as a physical shield from UV rays.

● *It gets you promoted*
According to leading image consultants, women who wear make-up at work are generally seen as more polished and up-to-date. Research shows that attractive people do better in interview situations, get better grades at school, are more likely to get more assistance from other people.

● *It improves your beauty habits*
Make-up wearers are more likely to follow a thorough cleansing routine, which not only removes the make-up but keeps the pores clear, and removes grime and pollution.

● *It makes you feel healthier*
Research has shown that women who take care of their appearance while ill have greater confidence and self-esteem than those who don't. Anecdotal accounts testify to the inspiriting, uplifting effect that beautifying with cosmetics has on hospital patients.

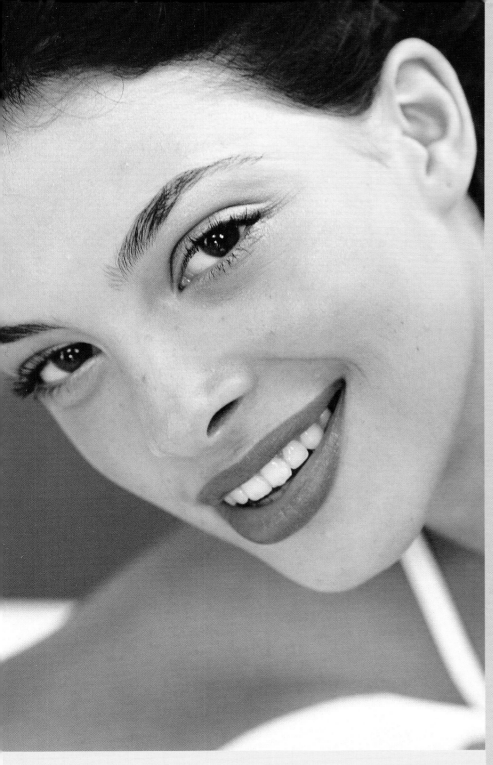

Instant glamour

This weekend is the ideal opportunity to brush up your glamour repertoire. Play around with colours and textures, and discover your own short cuts to glowing skin, sensuous lips and sexy eyes.

shortcuts to gorgeous looks

Skin

Intimate soirées call for immaculate skin. A thick layer of foundation is a cardinal sin, as are dolly-red cheeks. Instead think:

● natural

Choose a natural, dewy foundation, or use a sheer base only where you need it. Alternatively, a stick foundation is less messy and the texture works well with a cream blusher. Apply cream with fingers to the apple of the cheeks, then work outwards in small circles.

● flawless

To conceal a spot, blot your face with a tissue to remove excess oil. Using a shade of concealer that matches your skin tone or is one shade lighter, pat the colour over the spot, blending the edges with a cotton bud. Apply an oil-free liquid foundation, taking care not to rub over the concealer. A light dusting of powder patted over the spot will set the concealer and foundation.

● shimmery

Liven up your complexion with a rosy-toned blusher. Apply with a thick brush to the apple of the cheekbones, spiralling outwards, and to the brow bones and temples. Or apply a powder highlighter over the areas that catch the light – the forehead, nose, cheekbone and below the brow.

eyes

Even the 'windows to the soul' can be enhanced with a few sweeps of shade and colour. Try these strategies for totally entrancing, come-hither stares.

Big eyes

1 To make eyes look bigger, arch your eyebrows, either with a brow pencil or, if they are very unruly, by plucking (see page 83).

2 Apply a pale or neutral colour over the whole upper eye area, blending the outer edges.

3 Use a brown or grey eyeshadow (black can 'shrink' the eyes) from the middle to outer edges of the eye sockets. Start with just a little colour and gradually add more if needed. Blend well.

4 Brush a thin line of the darker shade into the lashes along the upper lid. Add a little shading under the eye at the outer edge, then apply highlighter underneath the outer brow line.

5 For the final touch, apply white pencil along the lower inner socket line of your eye, rubbing over with a cotton bud.

6 Curl your eyelashes, apply plenty of mascara and comb the lashes through with an eyelash definer. Voilà!

Golden eyes

1 Flatter an olive or dark skin with gold eyeshadow and berry-toned lipstick. Use your finger to apply gold cream shadow to the entire eye, keeping it intense on the lids and lightening it as you go up onto the brow bone.

2 Add a touch of gold shadow to the outer corners of the eyes and just under the lower lash line, to create a halo of gold around the eyes. Finish with a coat of black mascara. (To avoid hard lines, don't use eyeliner.)

3 Team with a berry-toned lip colour, and a gentle sweep of dark plum powder blusher.

Glossy eyes

1 To give your eyes glossy shine, combine slick, crisp colours such as green or sky blue. Using your ring finger, apply over the eyelids and brush a little along the lower lash lines.

2 To add a final shimmer, dab some lip balm over the top of your lids.

Fluttery eyes

1 Use a few false eyelashes to open up the eyes. For a feathery flutter, apply individual lashes of different lengths. Start on the outer corner of the eye with a medium-length lash, then apply a shorter one and work towards the middle of the eye, alternating between the two.

2 Make the eyes the focal point by coating your lips with a soft, shimmery, pink lipstick.

Sultry eyes

1 Sexy, smouldering eyes are always a winner, but the key is to keep it simple. Instead of eyeshadow, experiment with a light lip balm on your lids.

2 Apply a soft, black kohl liner to the outer corners of your top and bottom lids, extending it outwards slightly for a more dramatic effect.

3 As the focus is on your eyes, keep your lips natural. Just slick on some clear lipgloss with your fingers.

Sparkly eyes

1 Disco-diva eyes are easy to achieve. Slick petroleum jelly over the eyelids to act as a glue for glitter eyeshadow.

2 Apply glitter eyeshadow with a large, flat eyeshadow brush. Cover the lid, not the brow bone.

3 With such intense eyes you need to keep your foundation shine free, so use a light base, some concealer under the eyes, and a quick dusting of loose powder, with a sweep of soft, pinky blush over the cheeks.

4 Complement your dazzling eyes with a clear lip gloss and a dab of loose glitter on your cheeks. Then, simply sparkle!

hot lips

the fact that lipstick was strictly forbidden in certain oppressive eras in history makes it all the more seductive. Add to that the fact that painting one's lips red imitates the action of sexual arousal, and you have a good reason to give your lips the utmost attention...

The basics

● The key to long-lasting lip colour is careful preparation. Before applying lipstick, put petroleum jelly on your lips and blot well.
● Outline your lips with a lip pencil in a shade that matches your lipstick, or is just slightly lighter.
● Apply lipstick and blot with a tissue. Add another coat of lipstick. This should last for hours, because it has now stained the lips, especially if it's a dark shade.

Special lips

● Even the bare, 'no make-up' look requires effort. Prime your lips first, by very gently buffing them with a soft (baby's) toothbrush to remove any dry skin and boost the circulation. Then follow up with a good quality lip balm.
● Dark, glossy lips give a touch of instant glamour. Plum lip colour tends to suit everyone, especially blue-eyed blondes, as it really brings out their eye colour.
● Try this professional trick for textured lips: layer different shades and textures to create depth, intensity and original colour. If you're a redhead, try applying a layer of bronze gloss over terracotta lipstick.
● Sheer gloss suits every skin tone. For depth, use a neutral lip pencil first, smudging the colour inwards. Then add the gloss to the fullest part of the lips.

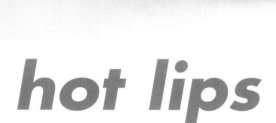

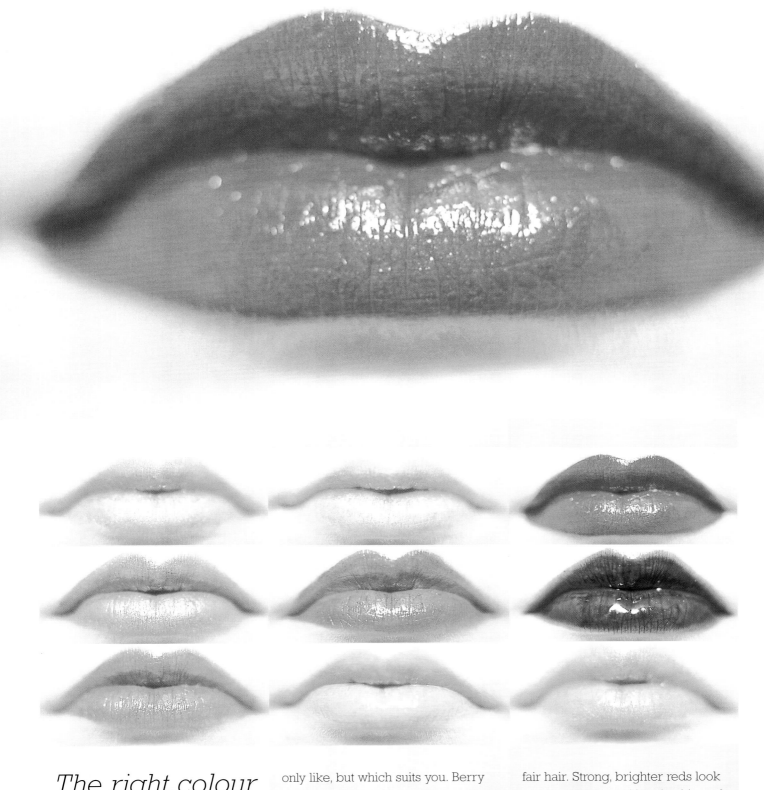

The right colour

● Finding a fabulous lipstick means choosing a shade which you not only like, but which suits you. Berry shades suit olive skins, while reds with pinkish undertones work best on those with fair complexions and fair hair. Strong, brighter reds look great on women with pale skin and dark hair, while deep, rich reds look stunning on dark skin.

Your glamourizing is now complete. All you need is a slinky dress, a splash of perfume, high heels and somewhere to party...

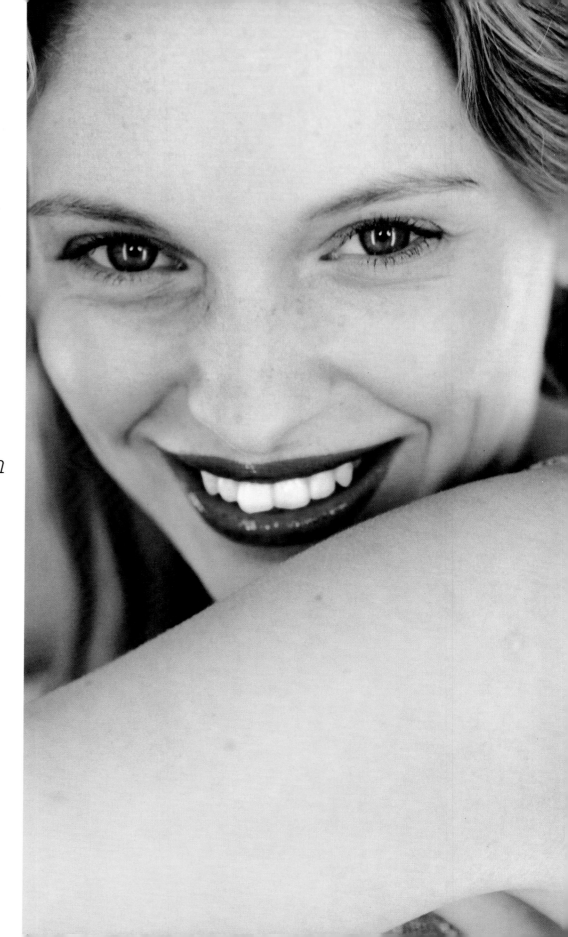

ACKNOWLEDGEMENTS

Thanks to Sèan Harrington, Managing director of Spa Resources and Elemis, and Noella Gabrielle, Director of Treatment Development for Elemis

For details of Elemis treatments (available at salons in the UK) and Aromapure products contact: Elemis Ltd, 57 The Broadway, Stanmore, Middlesex HA7 4DU
TEL: (+44) 020 8954 8033
FAX: (+44) 020 8954 7980

And also thanks to Susan Harmsworth, Founder and Chief Executive of ESPA, treatment and product range. For details of your nearest salon, product information and mail order contact: 01252 741600

NIA Workout
For more details of NIA workshops call 01444 461816 or email Helen Terry at Lhmotivation@earthlink.com

Walking story:
To contact your local Reebok walking instructor call 01524 591888

For more information on breathing exercises, read *Yoga for Stress* by Vimla Lalvani, published by Hamlyn

The yoga workout was designed exclusively for Zest by yoga expert Vimla Lalvani, who has produced yoga videos including *The Fountain of Youth*, *Yogacise* and *Yogacise II: The Body Beautiful*

Food programmes devised by Zest's nutrition expert, state-registered dietician Lyndel Costain

Recipes devised by Pat Alburey

And finally many thanks to Gloria Thomas, Suzanne Duckett, Karen Wheeler, Anita Bean, Sally Brown and Eve Cameron

BIBLIOGRAPHY

Beauty Wisdom by Bharti Vyas with Claire Haggard, published by Thorsons. Thorsons is an imprint of HarperCollins

The Book of Aromatherapy Blends by Christine Wildwood, published by HarperCollins

The Beauty Bible by Sarah Stacey and Josephine Fairley, published by Kyle Cathie

The Tropical Spa: Asian Secrets of Health, Beauty and Relaxation by Sophie Benge, published by Periplus

Spirit of the Home: How to Make Your Home a Sanctuary by Jane Alexander, published by Thorsons

PHOTOGRAPH CREDITS

1 Grand Illusions; 4 (top) Camera Press; 4 (bottom) National Magazine Co./Kimball Lorio; 6-7 (top) The Holding Co.; 6-7 (bottom) National Magazine Co./Elsa Hutton; 9 Camera Press/Axel Springer Verlag; 10 National Magazine Co./Daniel Farmer; 12-13 National Magazine Co./David Loftus; 15 Images Colour Library; 16-17 Elizabeth Whiting Assoc.; 17 Tony Stone Images/Ken Scott; 18-19 National Magazine Co./Kimball Lorio; 20 Descamps; 20-21 Tony Stone Images/Paul Webster; 22-23 National Magazine Co./David Loftus; 24-25 Tony Stone Images/Thomas Braise; 26-27 National Magazine Co./Daniel Ward; 28-29 (4 shots) National Magazine Co./Jason Bell; 30 National Magazine Co.; 31 Camera Press/Maureen Barrymore; 32-33 Tony Stone Images/Andre Perlstein; 33 (top) Camera Press/Richard Open;

33 (bottom) Camera Press/Lars Matzen; 34-35 Tony Stone Images/Deborah Jaffe; 36-37 National Magazine Co./Chris Lane; 38-39 Images Colour Library; 40-41 National Magazine Co./Barry Hollywood; 42-43 National Magazine Co./Daniel Ward; 44-47 (13 shots) National Magazine Co./Justin Quick; 48 National Magazine Co./Steve Wallis; 50-51 National Magazine Co./Tom Corbett; 52 Tony Stone Images; Ken Scott; 53 (top) Images Colour Library; 53 (centre) Images Colour Library; 53 (bottom) Images Colour Library; 54-55 National Magazine Co./Hugh Johnson; 56 (left) Paperchase; 56 (right) National Magazine Co./Jason Bell; 57 (left) National Magazine Co./Jason Bell; 57 (right) National Magazine Co./Jason Bell; 58-59 National Magazine Co./Anna Stevenson; 60-61 Tony Stone Images/David Roth; 62-63 (7 shots) National Magazine Co./Daniel Ward;

64 (bottom) Welbeck Golin/Harris Commincations/Grand Illusions; 64-65 National Magazine Co./Chris Kolk; 66-67 Elizabeth Whiting Assoc.; 68-71 (7 shots) National Magazine Co./Jason Bell; 72-73 Tony Stone Images/Mark Williams; 73 National Magazine Co./David Loftus; 74-75 National Magazine Co./Daniel Ward; 75 (top) Camera Press/Axel Springer Verlag; 75 (bottom) Camera Press/Axel Springer Verlag; 76 National Magazine Co./Heather Farel; 77 National Magazine Co.; 78 National Magazine Co./Ian Skelton; 79 National Magazine Co./Ian Skelton; 80-81 National Magazine Co./Tierney Gearon; 82 National Magazine Co./Tom Corbett; 83 (right) Camera Press/Shaz; 83 (inset) Camera Press/Berry; 84-85 National Magazine Co./Chris Kolk; 85 (6 shots) Images Colour Library; 86 National Magazine Co./Tim Brett-Day; 87 (3 shots) Images Colour Library; 88 National Magazine Co.;

89 National Magazine Co./Sergio Veranes; 91 National Magazine Co./Heather Farel; 92-93 (13 shots) National Magazine Co.; 94 National Magazine Co./Sergio Veranes

INDEX